POCKET ATLAS OF BODY CT ANATOMY

Second Edition

Pocket Atlas of Body CT Anatomy

Second Edition

W. Richard Webb, M.D.

Professor of Radiology
Chief, Thoracic Imaging
Department of Radiology
University of California San Francisco Medical Center
San Francisco, California

Michael B. Gotway, M.D.

Assistant Professor of Radiology
Director, Radiology Residency
Chief, Thoracic Imaging, San Francisco General Hospital
Department of Radiology
University of California San Francisco School of Medicine
San Francisco, California

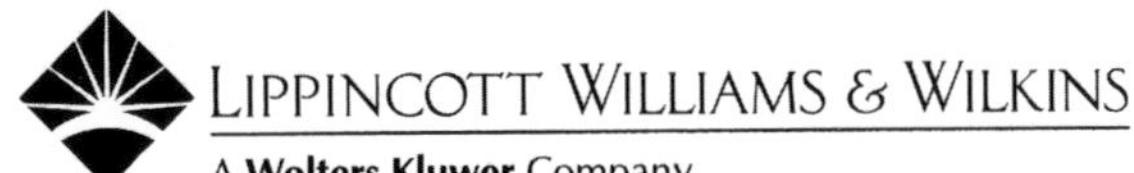

Philadelphia • Baltimore • New York • London
Buenos Aires • Hong Kong • Sydney • Tokyo

Acquisitions Editor: Joyce-Rachel John
Developmental Editor: Sara Lauber
Production Editor: Elaine Verriest McClusky
Printer: Strategic Content Imaging

530 Walnut Street
Philadelphia, PA 19106 USA
LWW.com

Printed in China

Library of Congress Cataloging-in-Publication Data

Webb, W. Richard (Wayne Richard), 1945–
Pocket atlas of body CT anatomy/W. Richard Webb, Michael B. Gotway.—2nd ed.
p. cm.
ISBN 13: 978-0-7817-3663-3
ISBN 10: 0-7817-3663-3
1. Tomography—Atlases. 2. Tomography—Handbooks, manuals, etc. I. Gotway, Michael B. II. Title
[DNLM: 1. Tomography, X-Ray Computed—Atlases. 2. Anatomy—Atlases. WN 17
W368p 2002]
QM25.W38 2002
611′.0022′2—dc21

2001050355

---

24 23 22 21

To Emma and Brett, whose delight in learning, and ignorance of CT anatomy, have been my inspiration.

To Clement, Patricia, and Mary Pat for their constant support and understanding.

Contents

Preface

This atlas is intended to provide a practical, anatomical guide to CT anatomy of the neck, thorax, abdomen, and pelvis. The structures identified are those of most importance in clinical body imaging.

The scans used for this atlas were obtained using spiral scanners capable of high-resolution volumetric imaging. The majority of images shown are axial views. Examples of relevant sagittal, coronal, and oblique plane reconstructions are also provided. Scans of the neck and thorax are each from a single patient. Scans of the abdomen and female pelvis are from a young woman; images of the male pelvis are also included.

Scans of the neck and thorax are 5 mm in thickness. At important levels in the thorax, both lung window (level –700 HU; width 1000 HU) and mediastinal window (level 40 HU; width 400 HU) images are shown. High-resolution CT images (1.25 mm thick) of the lung are also provided at selected levels.

Scans of the abdomen and pelvis are 7 mm thick. Abdominal scans were obtained during the "portal venous phase" of contrast enhancement, showing both arteries and veins. "Arterial phase" images through the upper abdomen (2.5 mm thick) are also included in order to show important arterial branches of the abdominal aorta.

W. Richard Webb, M.D.
Michael B. Gotway, M.D.

Abbreviations

ant = anterior
post = posterior
art = artery/arteries
pulm = pulmonary
seg = segment(s)
LLL = left lower lobe
LUL = left upper lobe
RLL = right lower lobe
RML = right middle lobe
RUL = right upper lobe

Neck and Larynx

scan level
(See image on page 12.)

1. mandible
2. tongue
3. pharynx
4. internal jugular vein
5. internal carotid art
6. external carotid art
7. external jugular vein
8. parotid gland

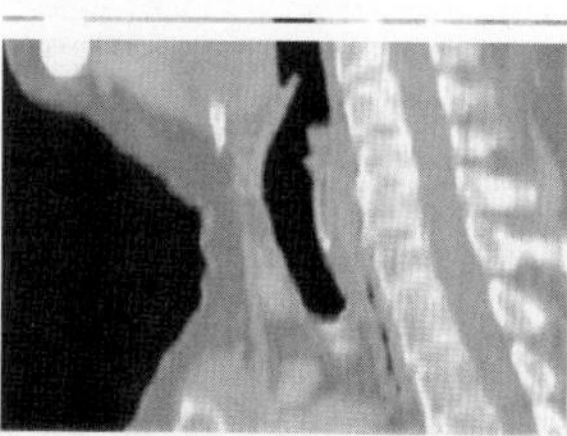

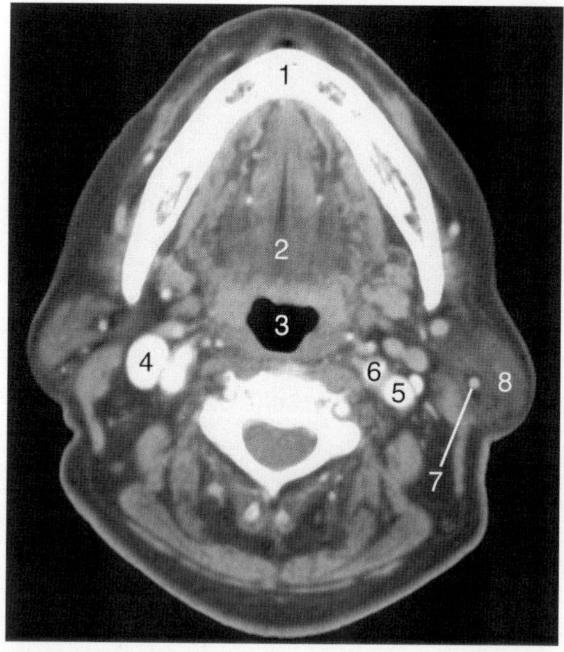

scan level
(See image on page 12.)

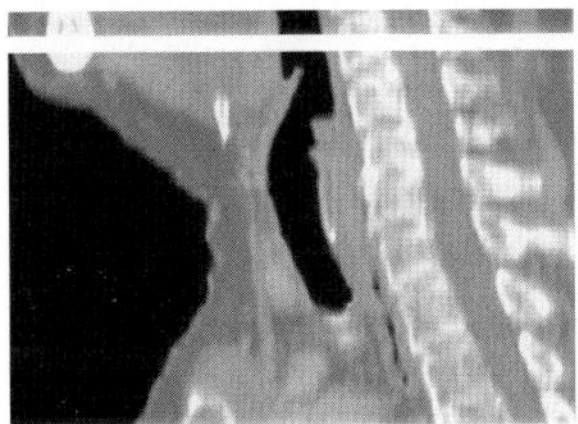

1. mandible
2. base of tongue
3. pharynx
4. internal jugular vein
5. common carotid art
6. sternocleidomastoid muscle
7. external jugular vein
8. vertebral art
9. vertebral body
10. posterior lamina

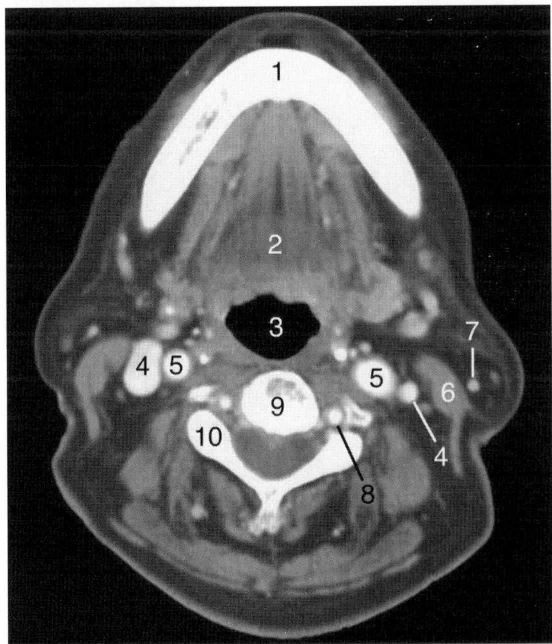

1. mandible
2. submandibular gland
3. epiglottis
4. internal jugular vein
5. common carotid art
6. sternocleidomastoid muscle
7. external jugular vein
8. greater cornu of hyoid bone

scan level
(See image on page 12.)

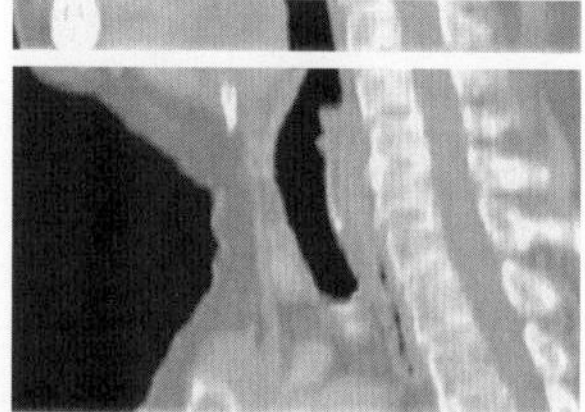

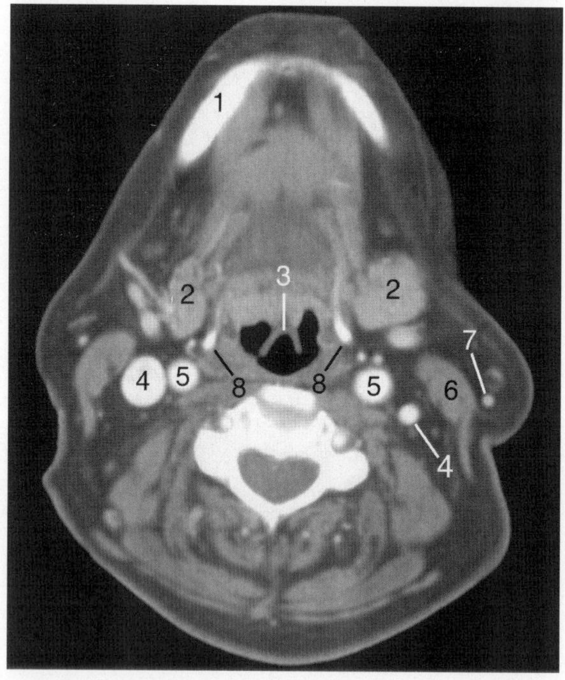

scan level
(See image on page 12.)

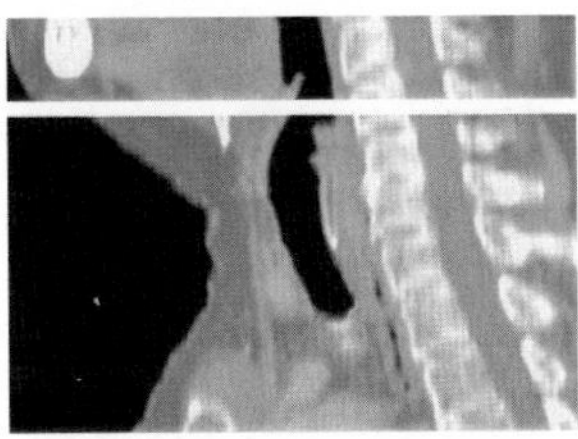

1. hyoid bone
2. vallecula
3. epiglottis
4. superior cornu thyroid cartilage
5. internal jugular vein
6. common carotid art
7. sternocleidomastoid muscle
8. submandibular gland

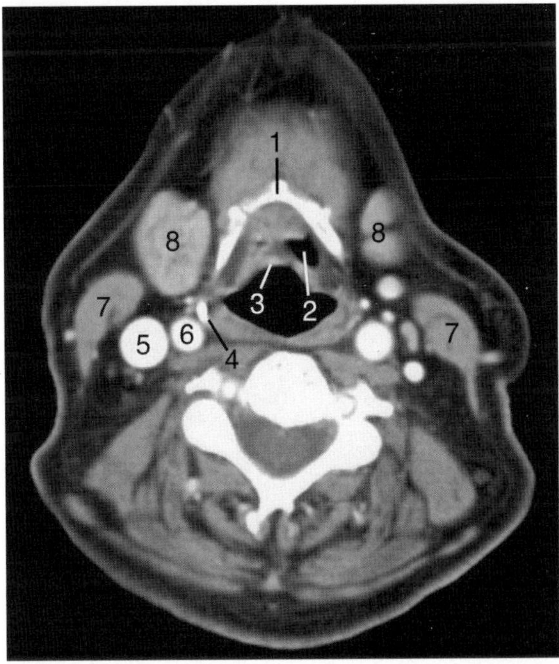

scan level
(See image on page 12.)

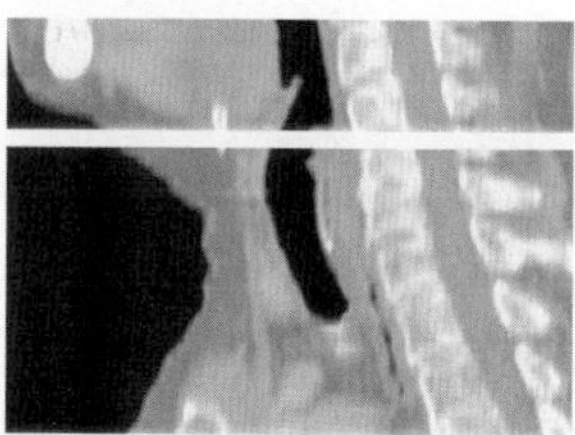

1. hyoid bone
2. thyroid cartilage
3. superior cornu thyroid cartilage
4. epiglottis
5. preepiglottic space
6. internal jugular vein
7. common carotid art
8. sternocleidomastoid muscle
9. pharyngeal constrictor muscles

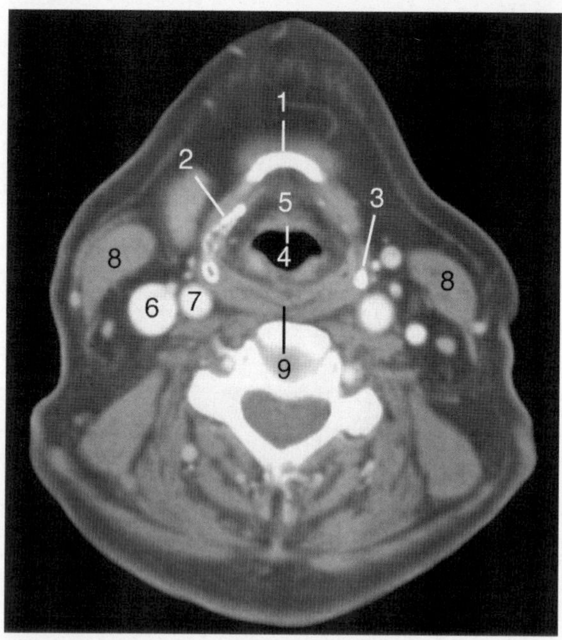

scan level
(See image on page 12.)

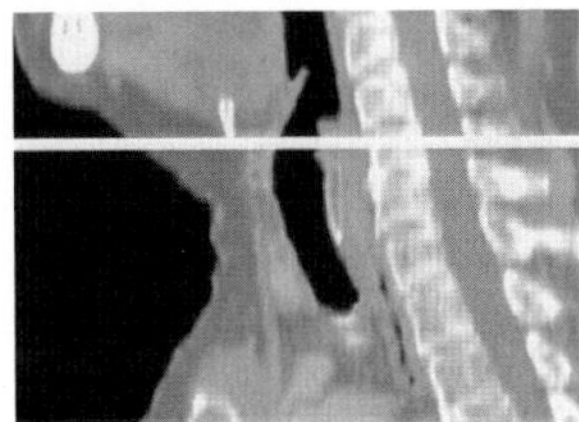

1. thyroid cartilage
2. laryngeal ventricle
3. aryepiglottic fold
4. pyriform sinus
5. laryngeal airway
6. pharyngeal constrictor muscles
7. internal jugular vein
8. common carotid art
9. sternocleidomastoid muscle
10. external jugular vein
11. vertebral body
12. vertebral art

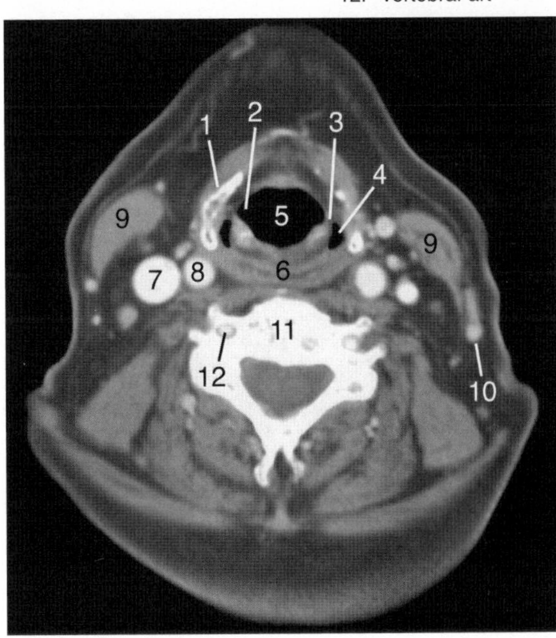

scan level
(See image on page 12.)

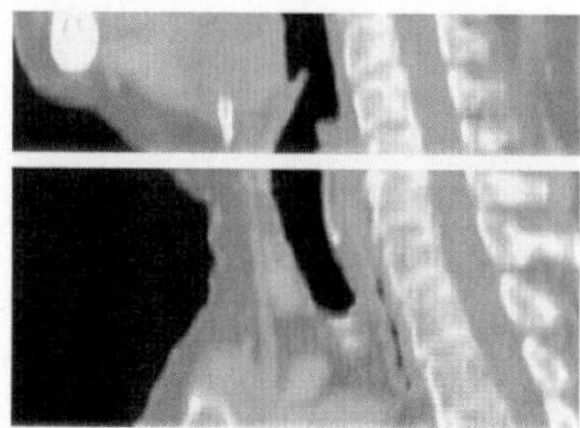

1. thyroid cartilage
2. cricoid cartilage
3. arytenoid cartilage
4. true vocal cord
5. ant commissure
6. laryngeal airway
7. internal jugular vein
8. common carotid art
9. sternocleidomastoid muscle
10. vertebral art
11. lymph node

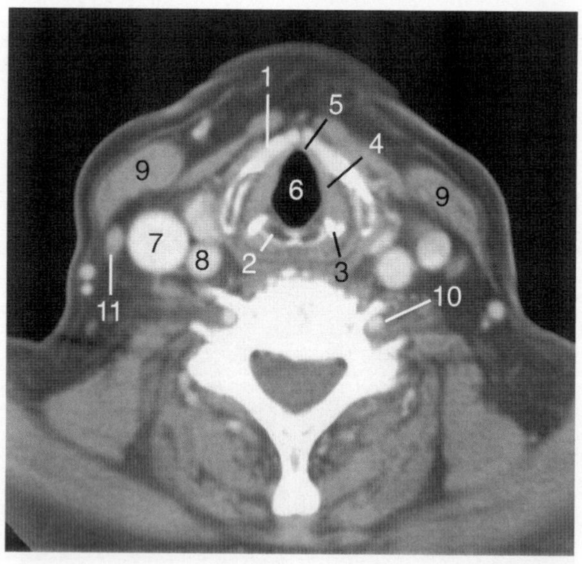

scan level
(See image on page 12.)

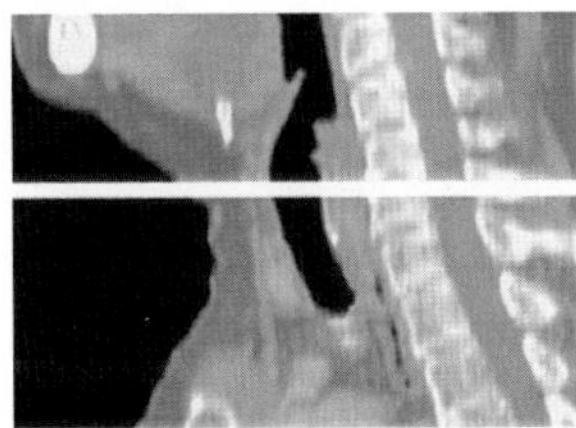

1. inferior cornu thyroid cartilage
2. cricoid cartilage
3. tracheal lumen
4. thyroid gland
5. internal jugular vein
6. common carotid art
7. sternocleidomastoid muscle
8. vertebral art

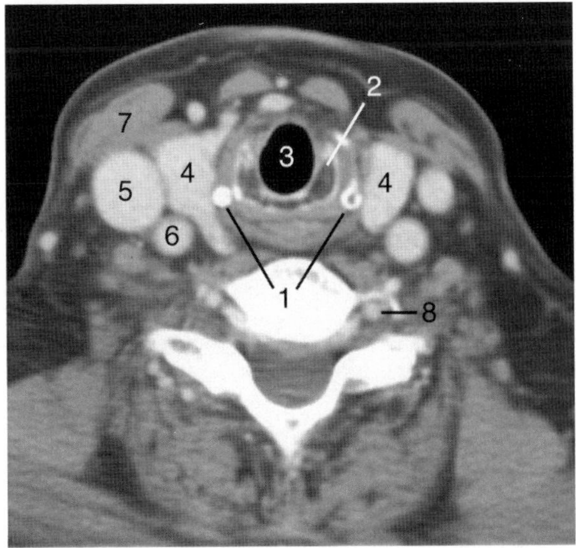

scan level
(See image on page 12.)

1. tracheal ring
2. tracheal lumen
3. post tracheal membrane
4. esophagus
5. thyroid gland
6. internal jugular vein
7. common carotid art
8. vertebral art
9. ant scalene muscle
10. middle and post scalene muscles
11. nerve root (brachial plexus)

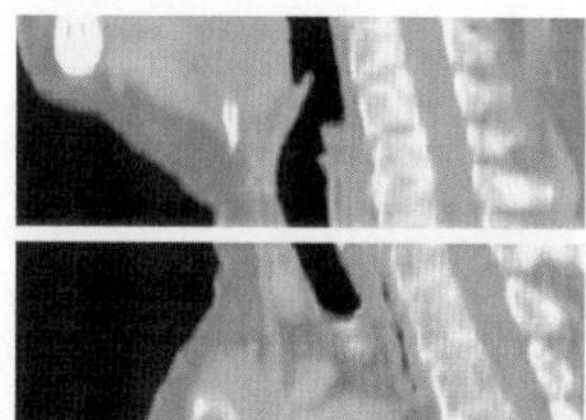

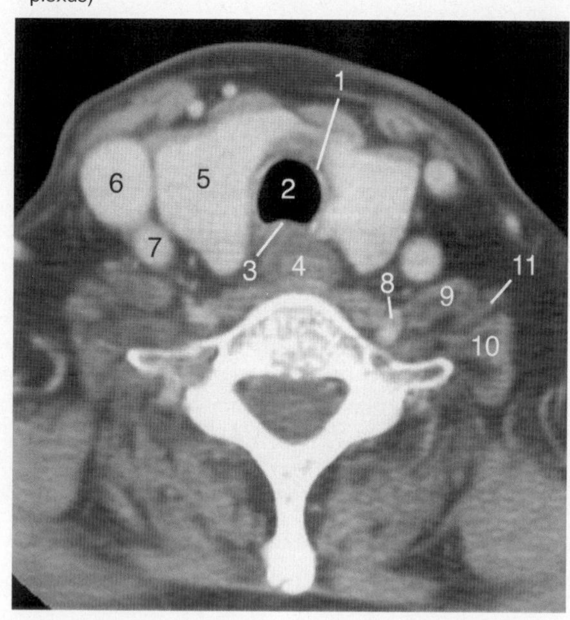

scan level
(See image on page 12.)

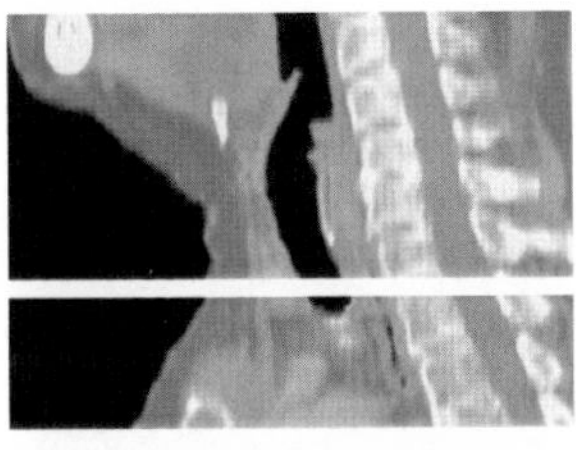

1. tracheal lumen
2. thyroid gland
3. thyroid isthmus
4. esophagus
5. internal jugular vein
6. common carotid art
7. vertebral art
8. ant scalene muscle
9. middle and post scalene muscles

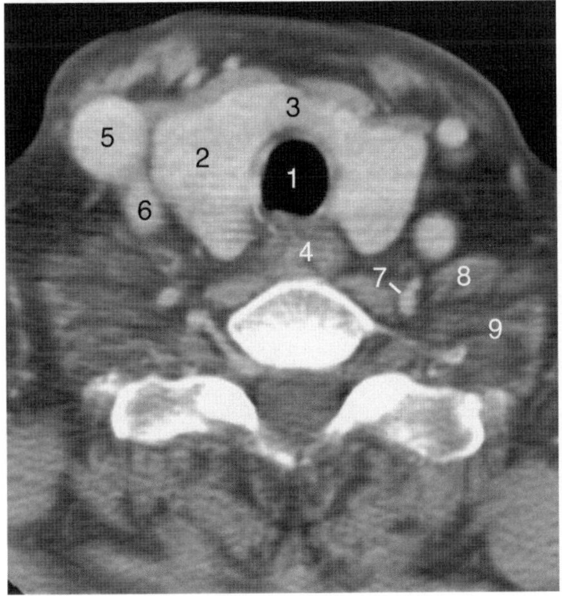

Neck and Larynx/Sagittal

scan level
(See image on page 8.)

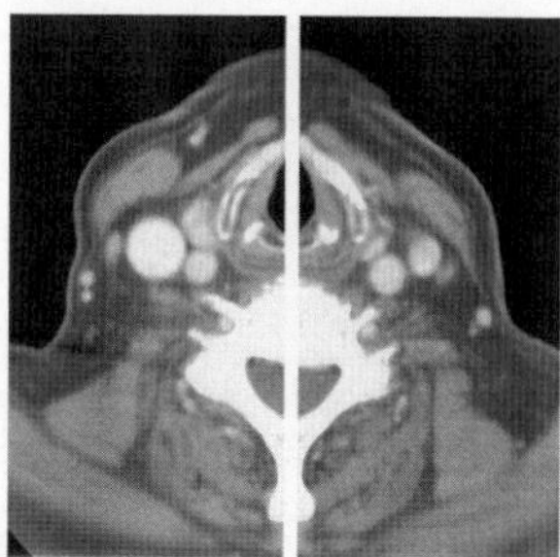

1. mandible
2. base of tongue
3. hyoid bone
4. epiglottis
5. preepiglottic space
6. vallecula
7. false vocal cord
8. laryngeal ventricle
9. true vocal cord
10. cricoid cartilage
11. tracheal lumen
12. esophagus
13. spinal canal
14. manubrium

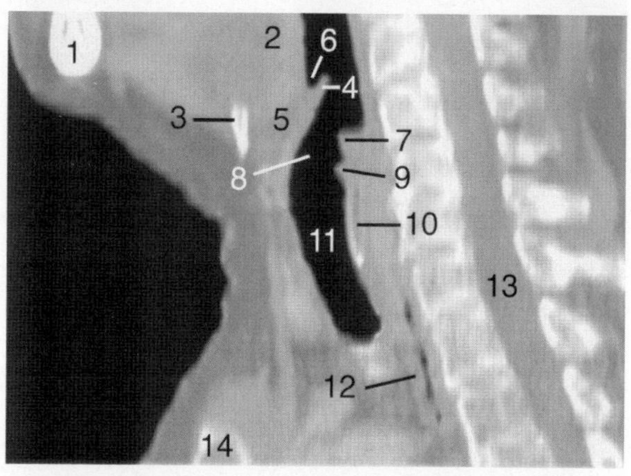

scan level
(See image on page 12.)

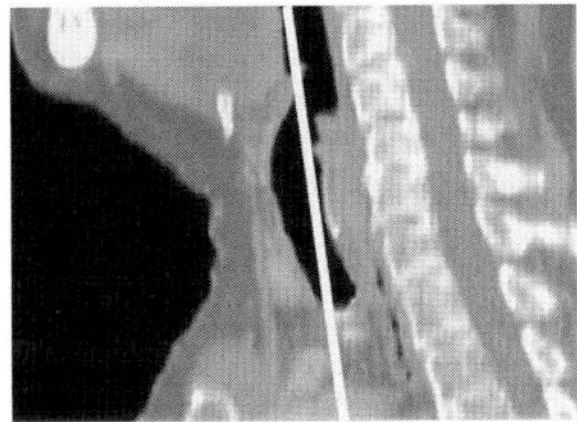

1. pharynx
2. epiglottis
3. aryepiglottic fold
4. hyoid bone
5. false vocal cord
6. laryngeal ventricle
7. true vocal cord
8. tracheal lumen
9. thyroid gland
10. carotid art
11. internal jugular vein

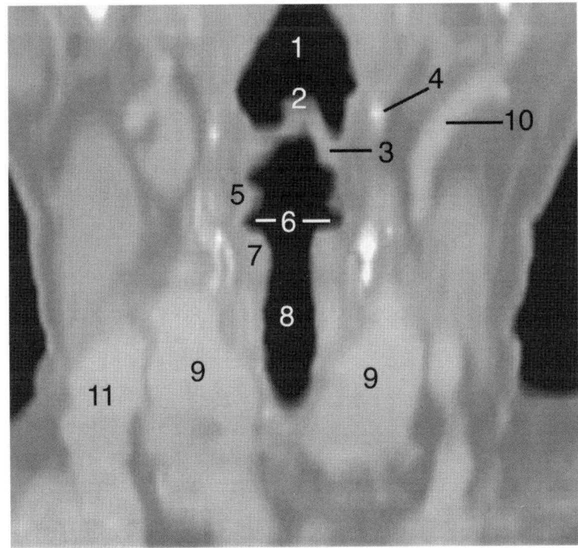

Thorax

scan level
(See image on page 51.)

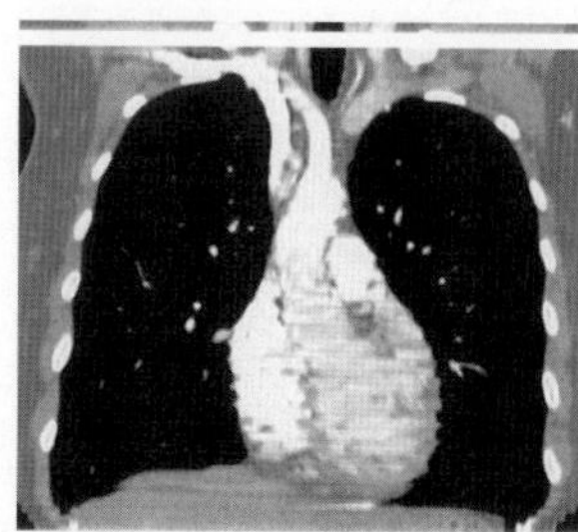

Mediastinal Window

1. thyroid gland
2. trachea
3. internal jugular vein
4. common carotid art
5. esophagus
6. vertebral art
7. clavicle
8. first rib
9. scapula

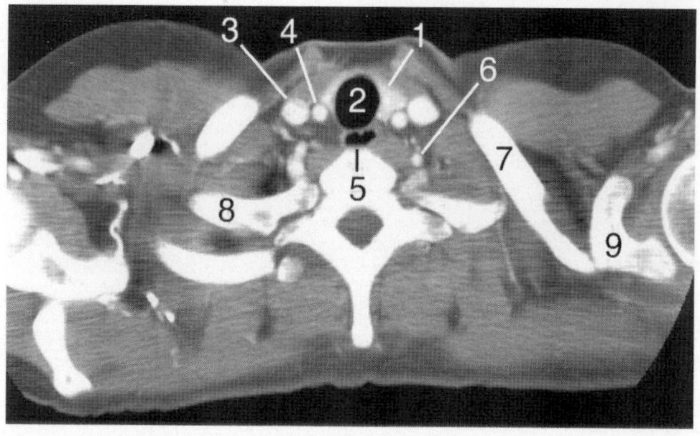

scan level
(See image on page 51.)

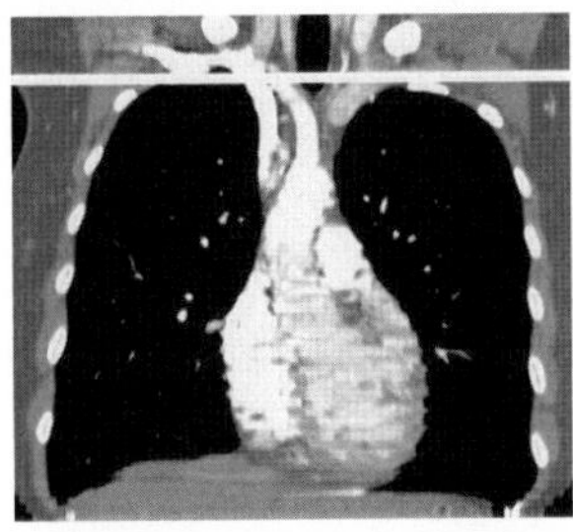

Mediastinal Window

1. trachea
2. common carotid art
3. internal jugular vein
4. lung apex
5. subclavian art
6. subclavian vein
7. clavicle
8. first rib
9. scapula (glenoid)

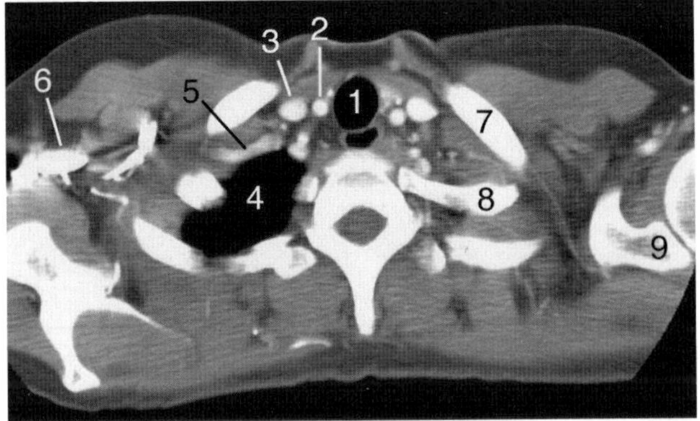

scan level
(See image on page 51.)

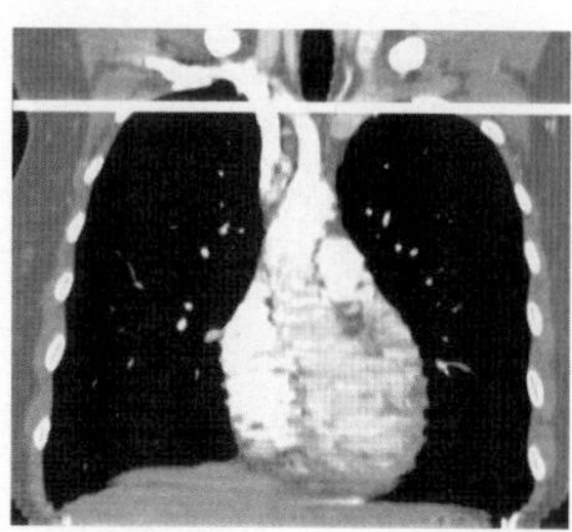

Mediastinal Window

1. trachea
2. esophagus
3. right common carotid art
4. head of clavicle
5. subclavian vein
6. right subclavian art
7. left vertebral art
8. left subclavian art
9. left subclavian (axillary) art
10. internal jugular vein
11. left common carotid art

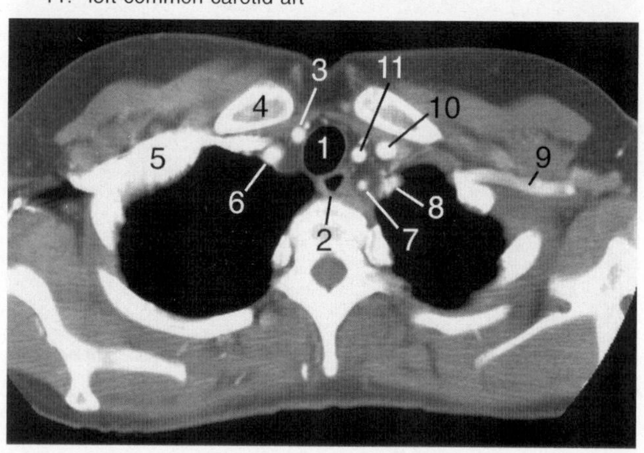

scan level
(See image on page 51.)

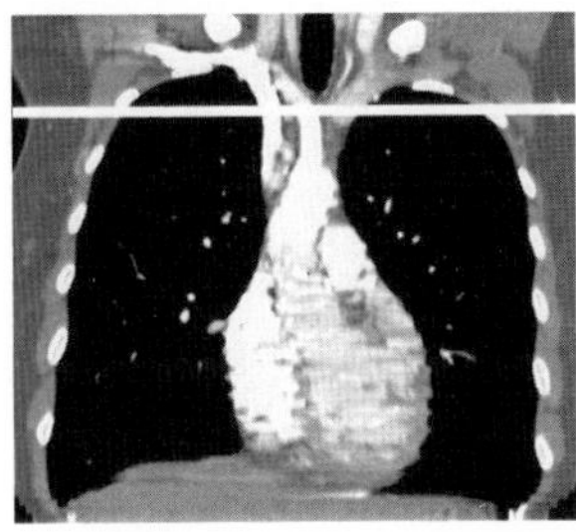

Mediastinal Window

1. trachea
2. right common carotid art
3. right subclavian art
4. right brachiocephalic vein
5. left subclavian art
6. left common carotid art
7. left brachiocephalic vein
8. subclavian vein (unopacified)
9. subclavian art
10. pectoralis major muscle
11. pectoralis minor muscle

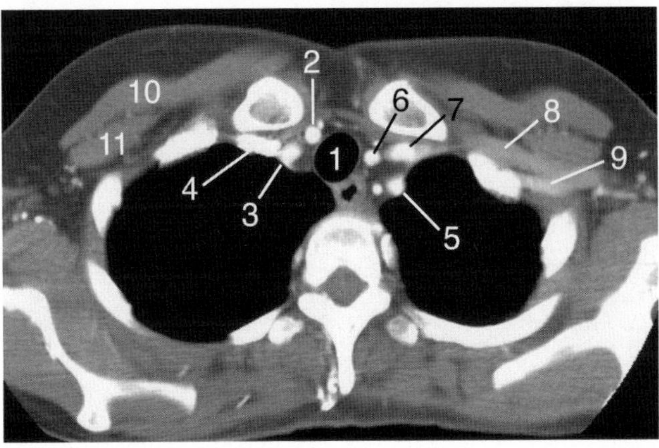

scan level
(See image on page 51.)

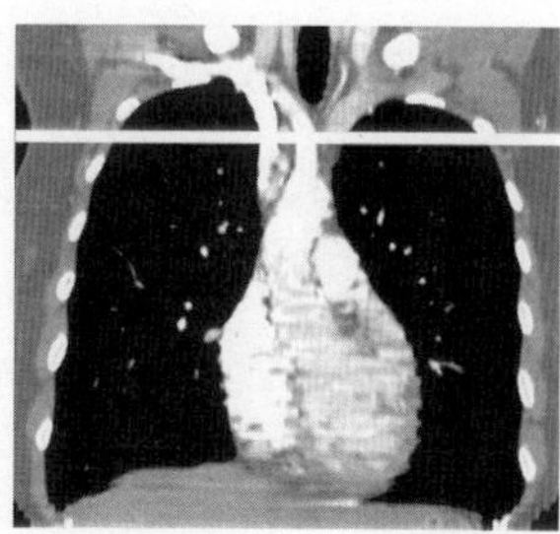

Mediastinal Window

1. trachea
2. esophagus
3. innominate art
4. right brachiocephalic vein
5. left brachiocephalic vein
6. left common carotid art
7. left subclavian art
8. manubrium
9. head of clavicle
10. axillary nodes and vessels

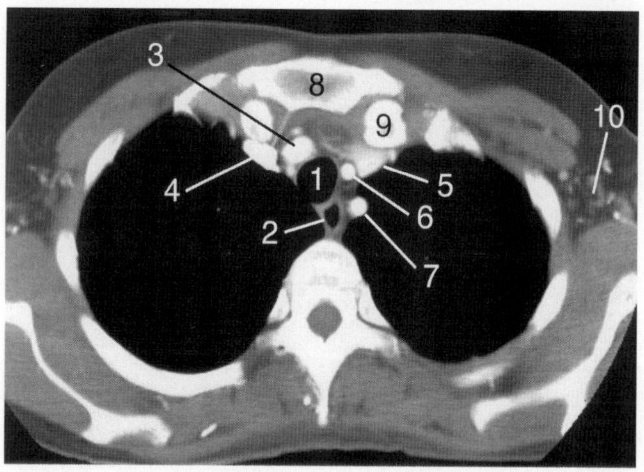

scan level
(See image on page 51.)

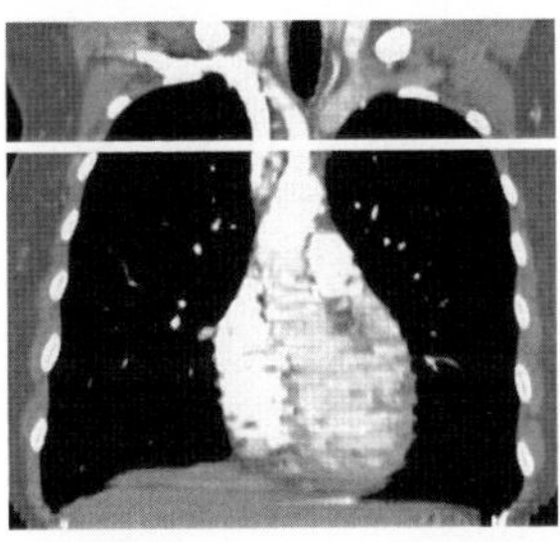

Mediastinal Window

1. trachea
2. esophagus
3. innominate art
4. right brachiocephalic vein
5. left brachiocephalic vein
6. left common carotid art
7. left subclavian art
8. normal lymph node

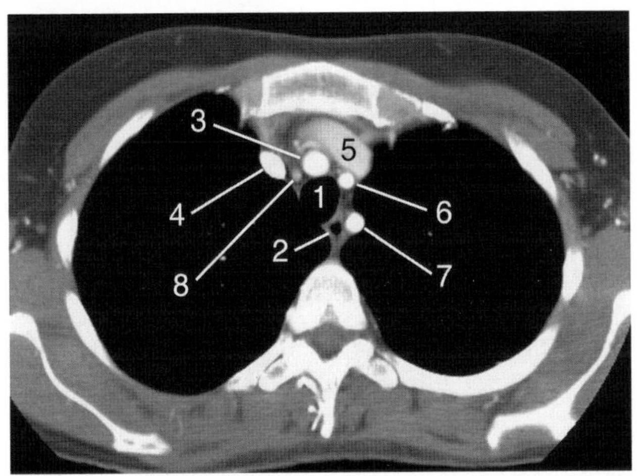

scan level
(See image on page 51.)

Mediastinal Window

1. trachea
2. esophagus
3. right brachiocephalic vein
4. left brachiocephalic vein
5. innominate art
6. left common carotid art
7. left subclavian art
8. thymus (left lobe)

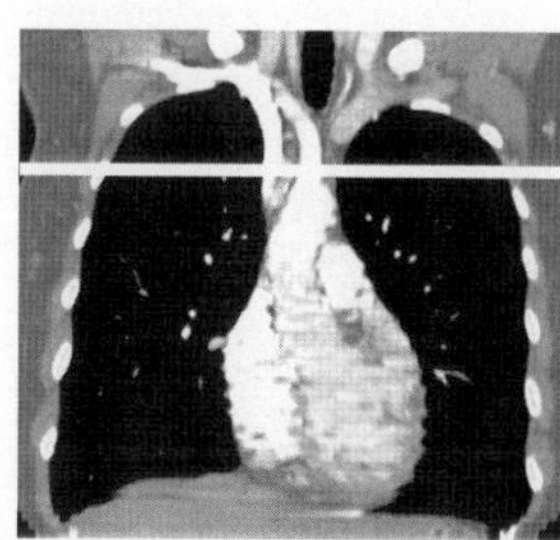

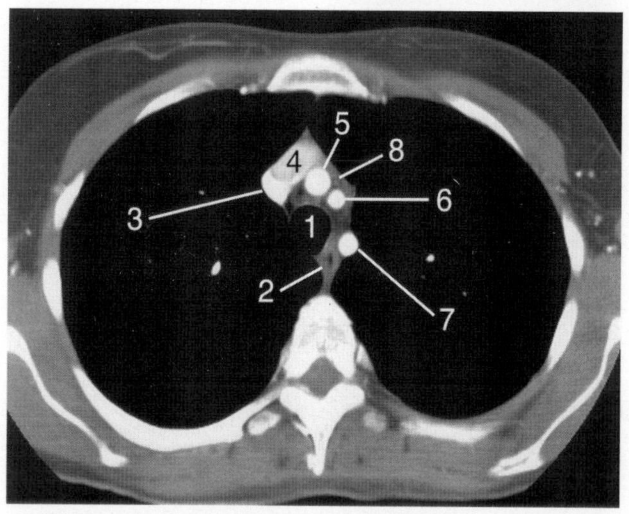

scan level
(See image on page 51.)

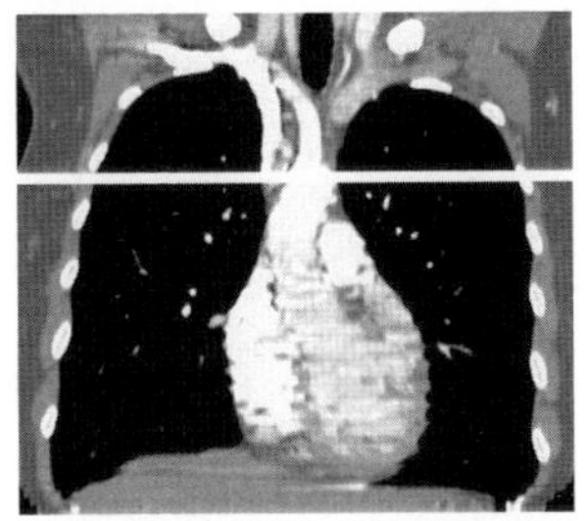

Mediastinal Window

1. trachea
2. esophagus
3. superior vena cava
4. internal mammary art
5. thymus
6. aortic arch

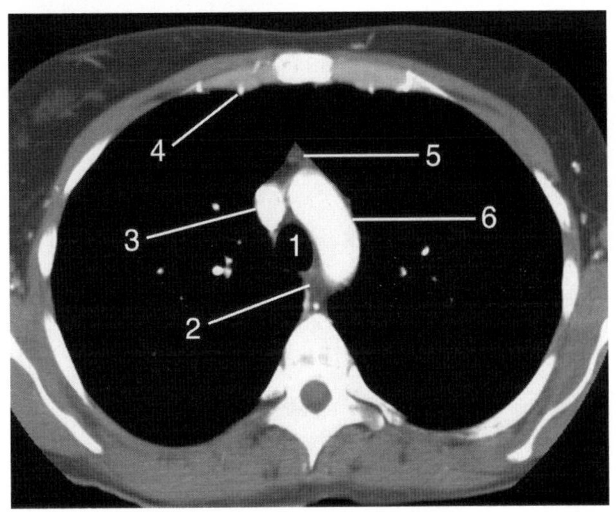

scan level
(See image on page 51.)

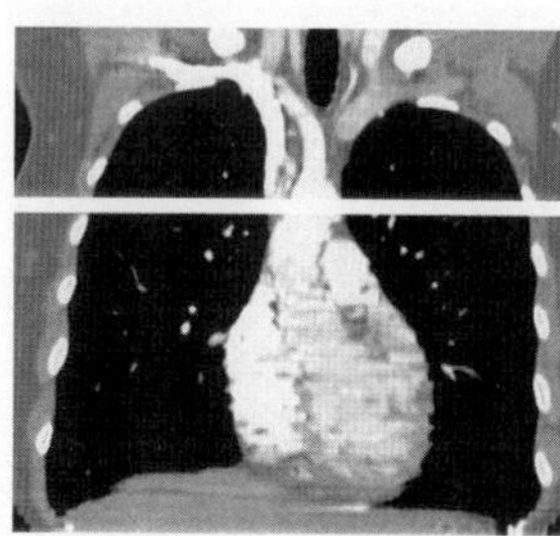

Mediastinal Window
1. trachea
2. superior vena cava
3. arch of azygos vein
4. internal mammary art
5. internal mammary vein
6. thymus
7. aortic arch
8. neural foramen

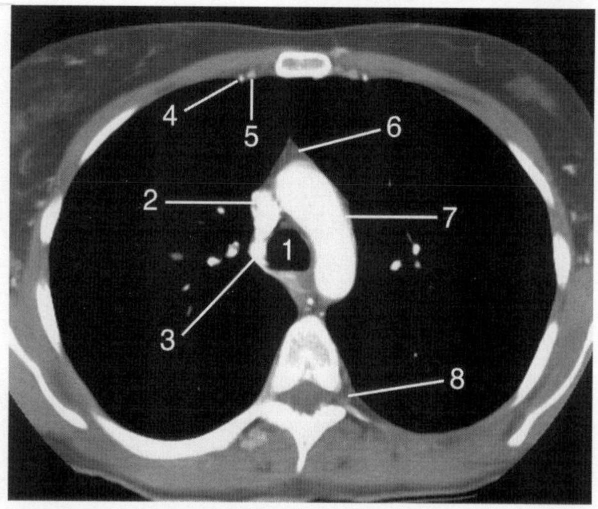

Same level as facing page.

scan level
(See image on page 50.)

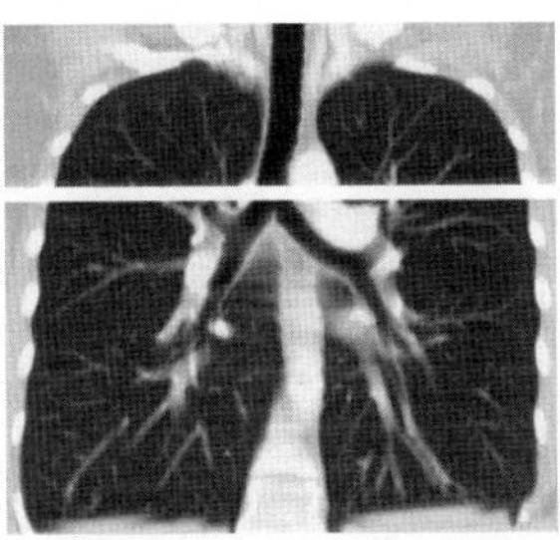

Lung Window

1. trachea
2. apical seg RUL bronchus
3. post seg RUL bronchus
4. apical-posterior seg LUL bronchus
5. major fissure
6. upper lobe
7. superior seg lower lobe

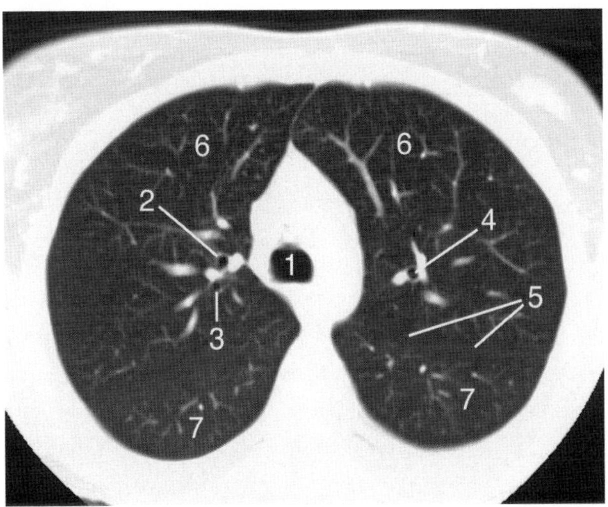

Same level as facing page.

scan level
(See image on page 51.)

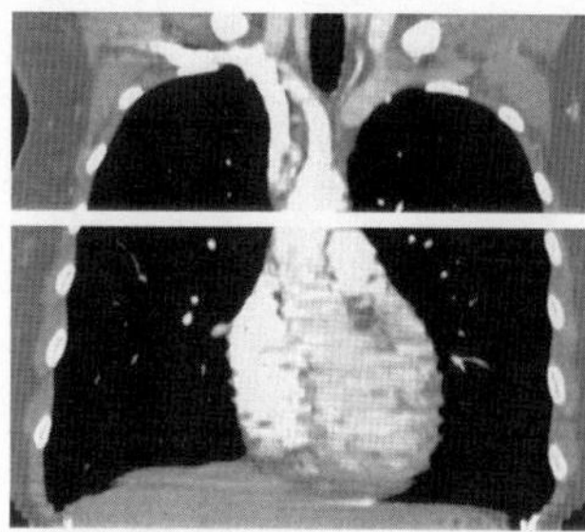

Mediastinal Window

1. tracheal carina
2. ascending aorta
3. descending aorta
4. superior aspect left pulm art
5. superior pericardial recesses
6. thymus
7. superior vena cava
8. truncus ant (RUL art)
9. normal lymph node
10. esophagus
11. azygos vein

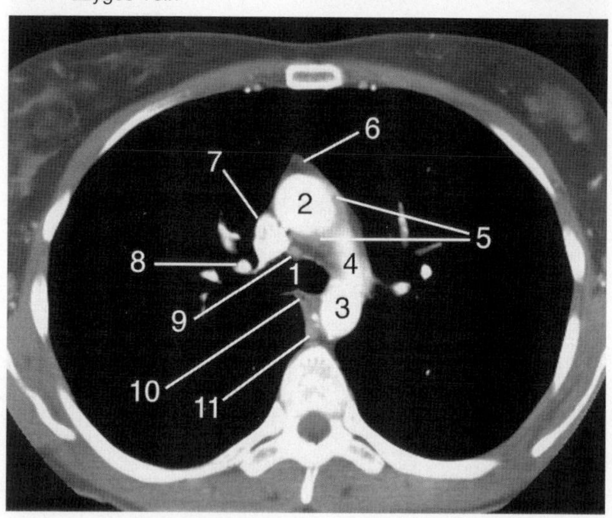

Same level as facing page.

scan level
(See image on page 50.)

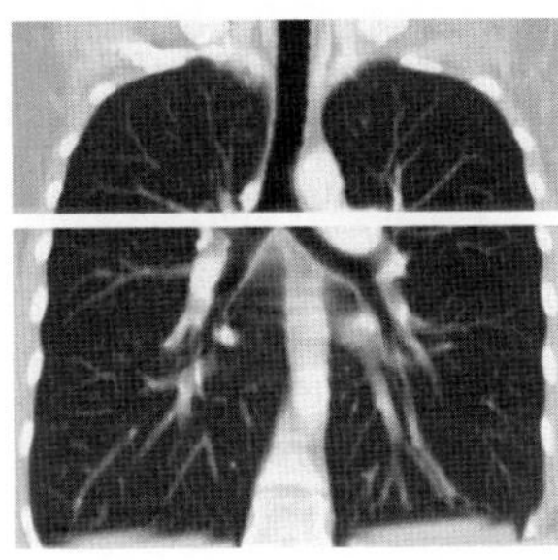

Lung Window

1. right main bronchus
2. tracheal carina
3. left main bronchus
4. RUL bronchus
5. post seg RUL bronchus
6. post vein RUL
7. ant seg RUL bronchus
8. ant seg RUL art
9. truncus ant (RUL art)
10. apical-posterior seg LUL bronchus
11. LUL art
12. pulm vein
13. ant junction line

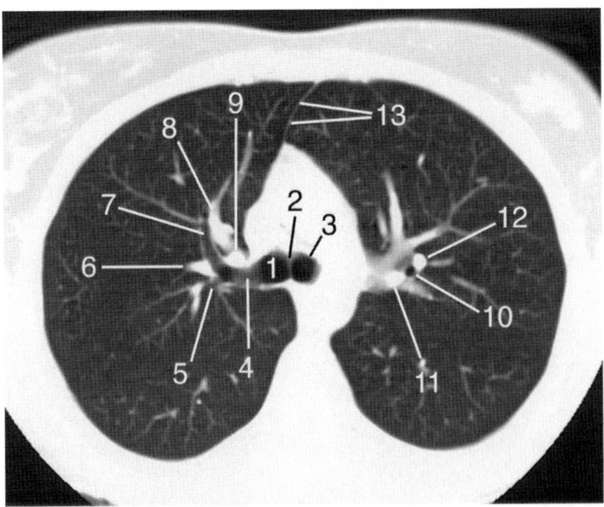

Same level as facing page.

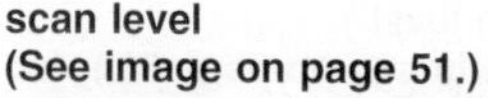
scan level
(See image on page 51.)

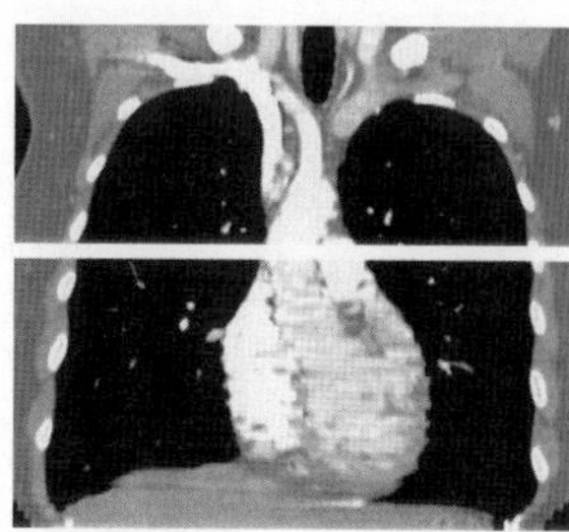

Mediastinal Window

1. ascending aorta
2. descending aorta
3. main pulm art
4. left pulm art
5. right pulm art
6. superior vena cava
7. left main bronchus
8. esophagus
9. normal subcarinal lymph node
10. superior pulm veins
11. azygos vein
12. hemiazygos vein branch
13. thymus

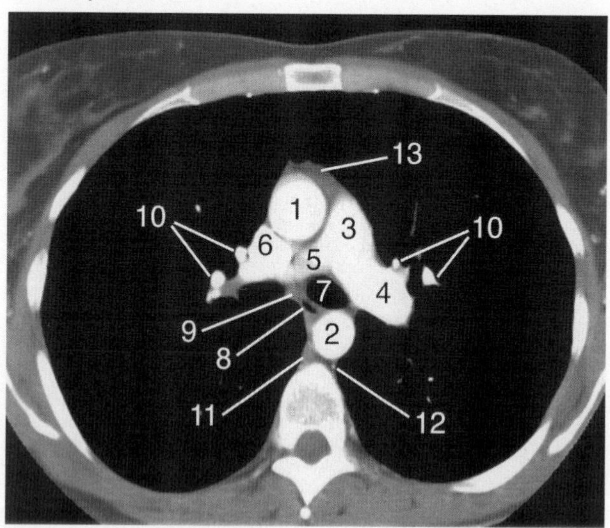

Same level as facing page.

scan level
(See image on page 50.)

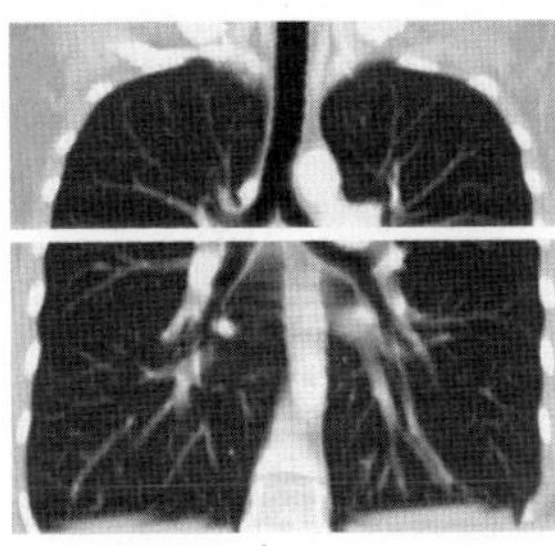

Lung Window

1. bronchus intermedius
2. left main bronchus
3. ant seg LUL bronchus
4. apical-posterior seg LUL bronchus
5. major fissure
6. minor fissure
7. ant junction line
8. RUL
9. RML
10. RLL

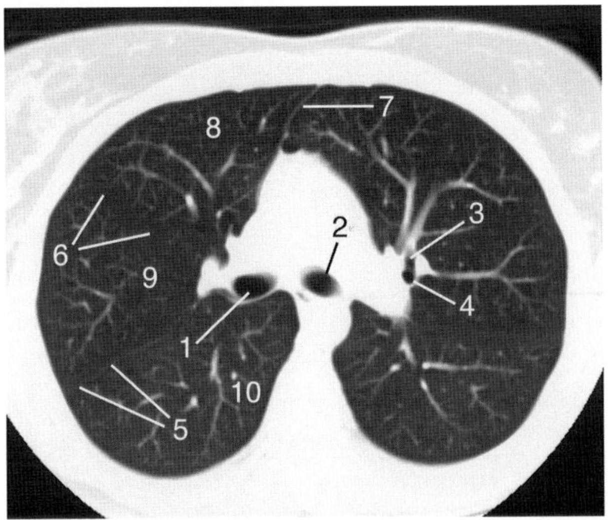

Same level as facing page.

scan level
(See image on page 51.)

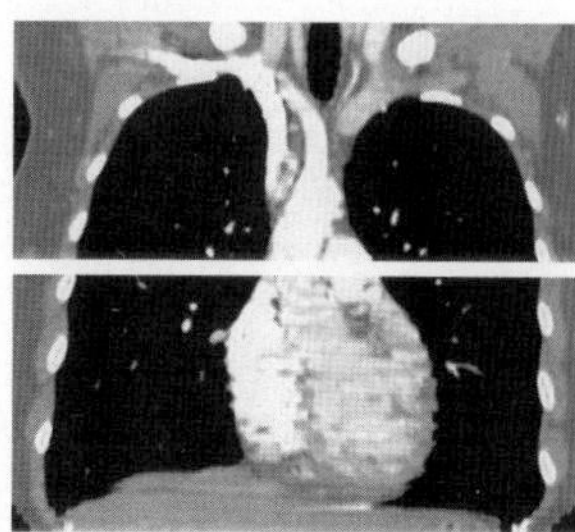

Mediastinal Window

1. ascending aorta
2. descending aorta
3. main pulm art
4. right pulm art
5. superior vena cava
6. interlobar pulm art
7. superior pulm vein
8. LUL bronchus
9. left main bronchus
10. bronchus intermedius
11. azygos vein

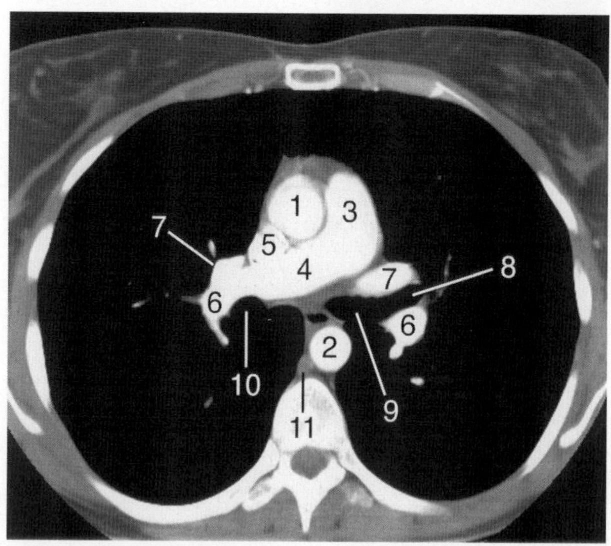

Same level as facing page.

scan level
(See image on page 50.)

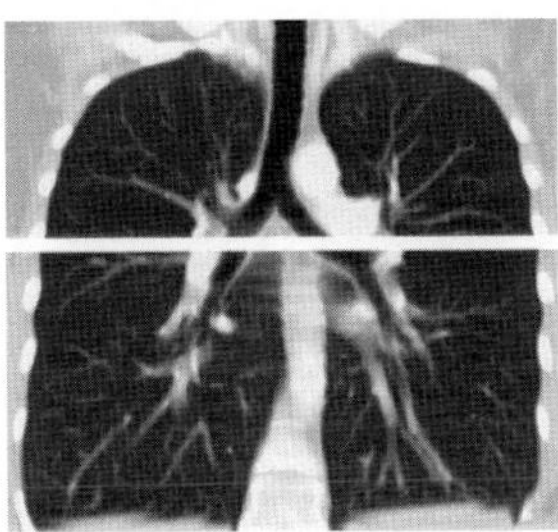

Lung Window

1. left main bronchus
2. LUL bronchus
3. bronchus intermedius
4. esophagus
5. interlobar pulm art

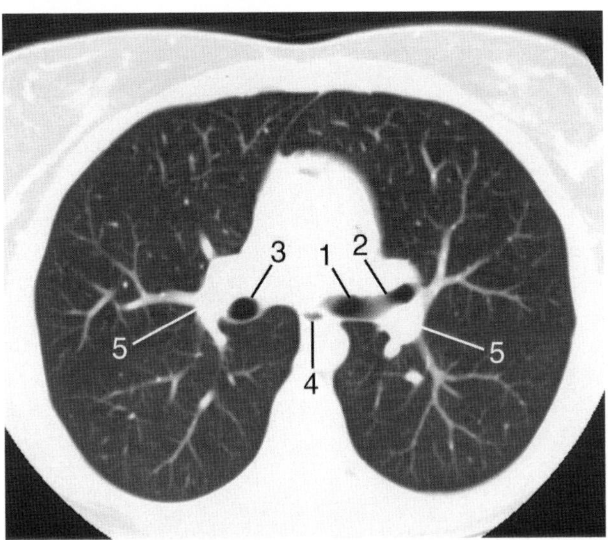

Same level as facing page.

scan level
(See image on page 51.)

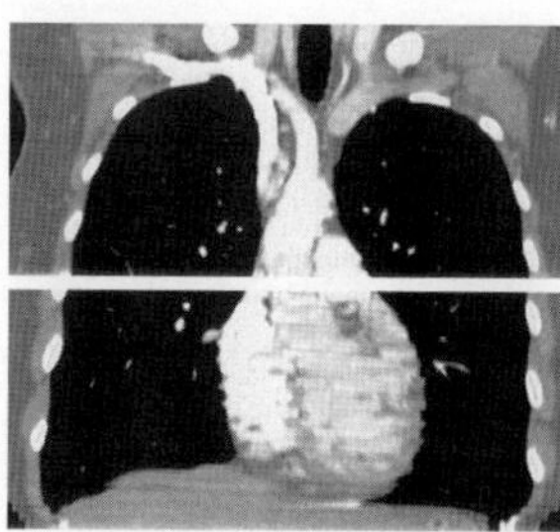

Mediastinal Window

1. ascending aorta
2. descending aorta
3. main pulm art
4. right pulm art
5. interlobar pulm art
6. superior pulm vein
7. right atrial appendage
8. lingular art

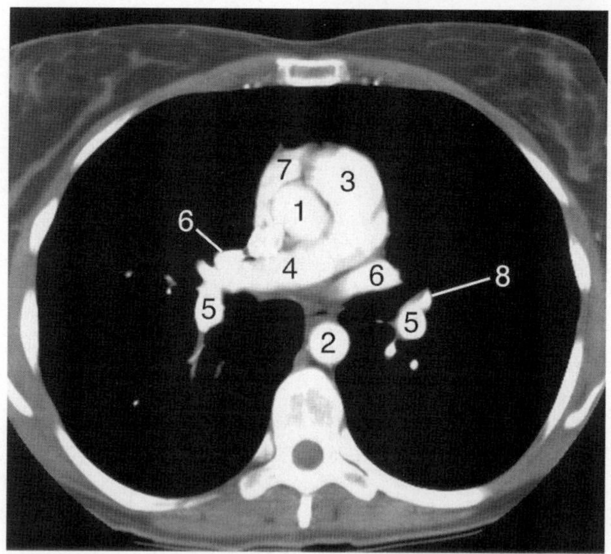

Same level as facing page.

scan level
(See image on page 50.)

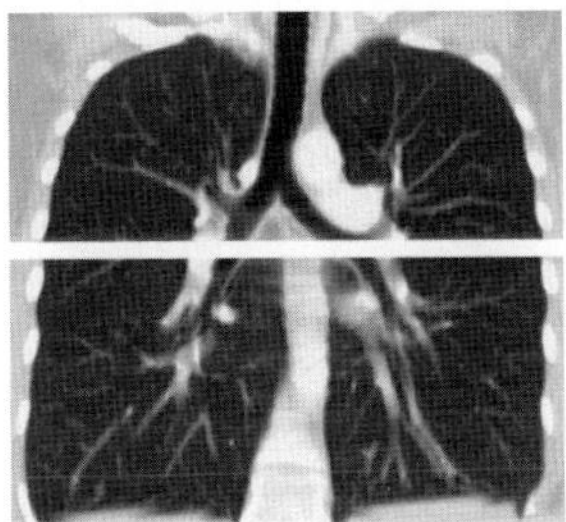

Lung Window

1. interlobar pulm art
2. superior pulm vein
3. bronchus intermedius
4. left main bronchus
5. LUL bronchus
6. lingular bronchus
7. superior lingular seg bronchus

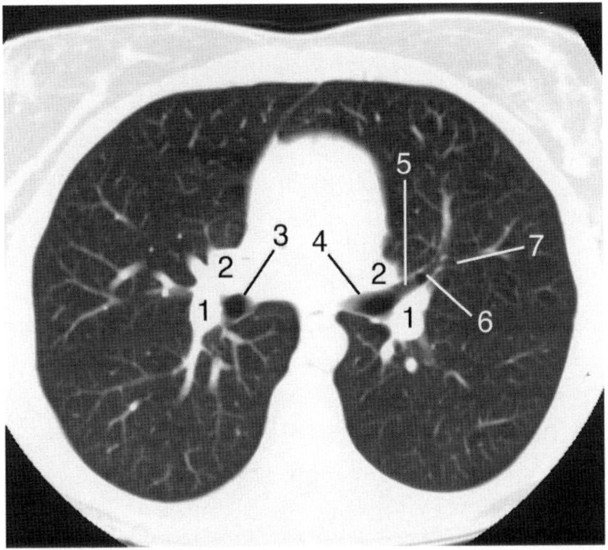

Same level as facing page.

scan level
(See image on page 51.)

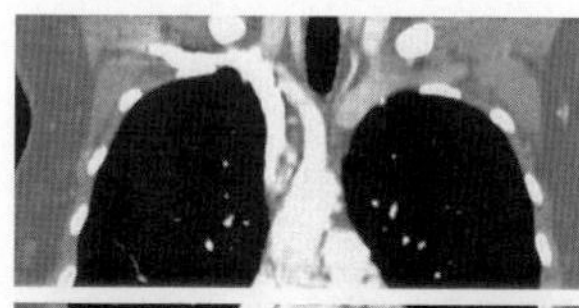

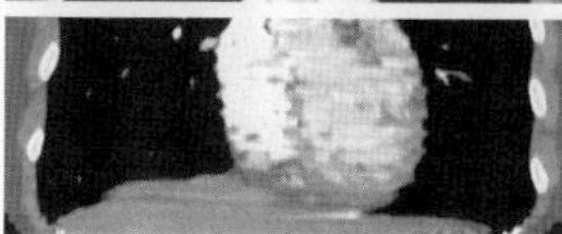

Mediastinal Window

1. ascending aorta
2. descending aorta
3. main pulm art
4. right atrium
5. right atrial appendage
6. superior pulm vein
7. lower lobe pulm art
8. RML art
9. lingular art
10. superior seg lower lobe art
11. azygos vein

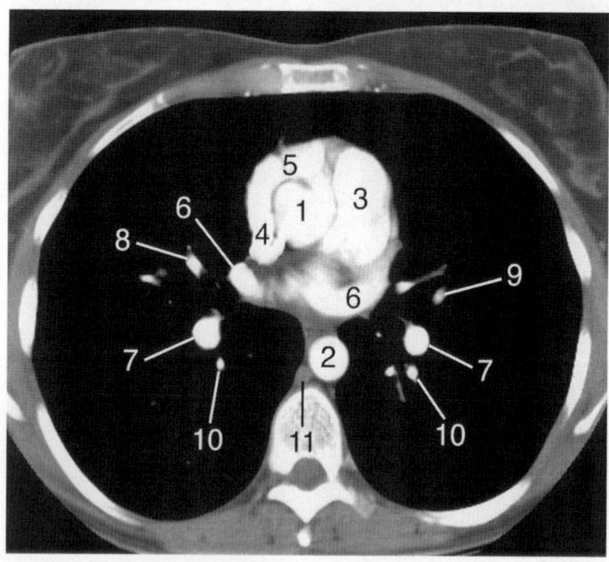

Same level as facing page.

scan level
(See image on page 50.)

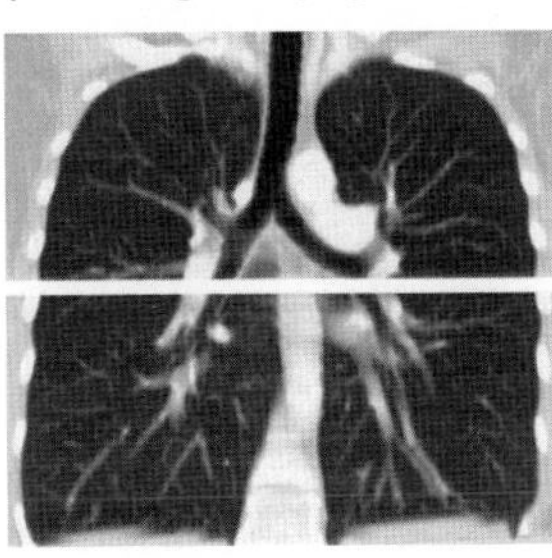

Lung Window

1. lower lobe pulm art
2. lower lobe bronchus
3. superior seg lower lobe bronchus
4. RML bronchus
5. medial seg RML bronchus
6. lateral seg RML bronchus
7. medial seg RML art
8. inferior seg lingula bronchus
9. inferior seg lingula art
10. lingular vein
11. superior seg lower lobe art

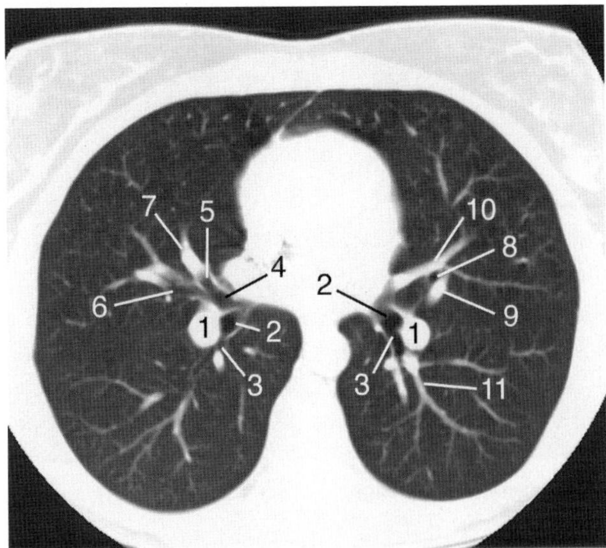

Same level as facing page.

scan level
(See image on page 51.)

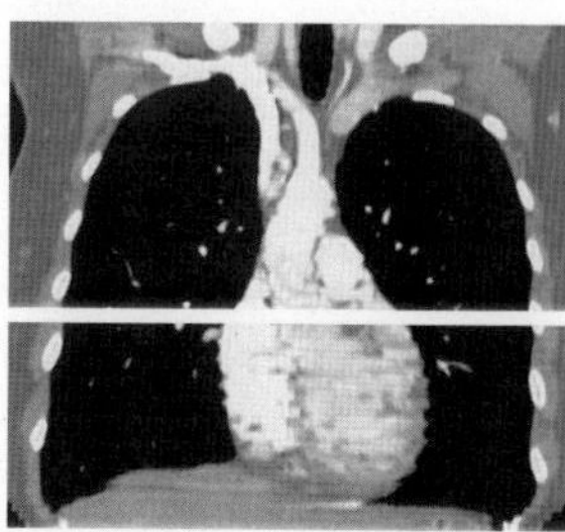

Mediastinal Window

1. ascending aorta
2. descending aorta
3. right ventricular outflow tract
4. right atrium
5. right atrial appendage
6. left atrium
7. left atrial appendage
8. basal lower lobe art
9. esophagus
10. left coronary art

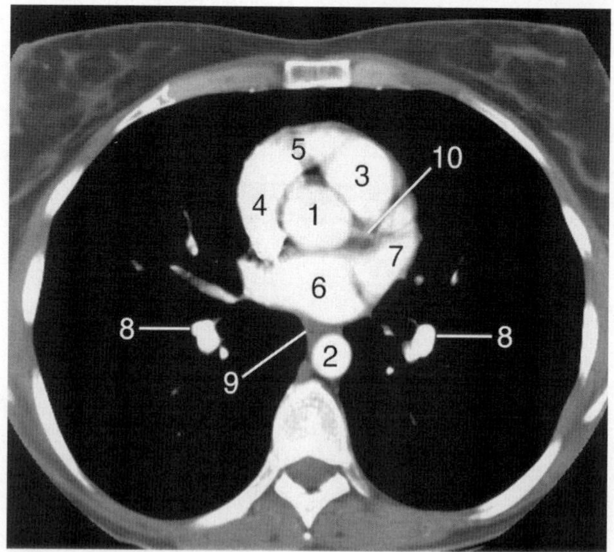

Same level as facing page.

scan level
(See image on page 50.)

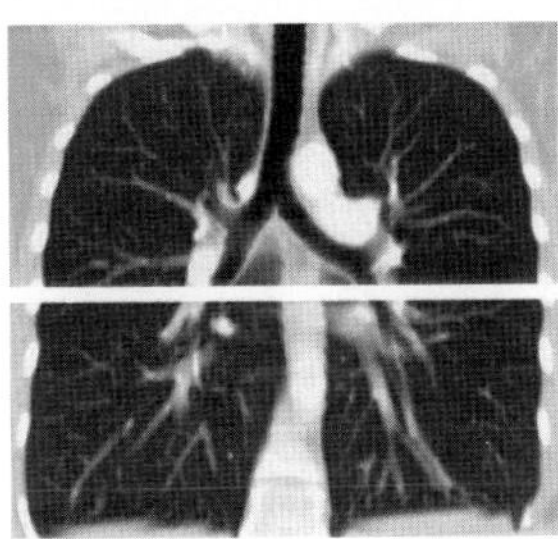

Lung Window

1. basal trunk lower lobe bronchus
2. basal lower lobe art
3. RML vein
4. medial seg RML art

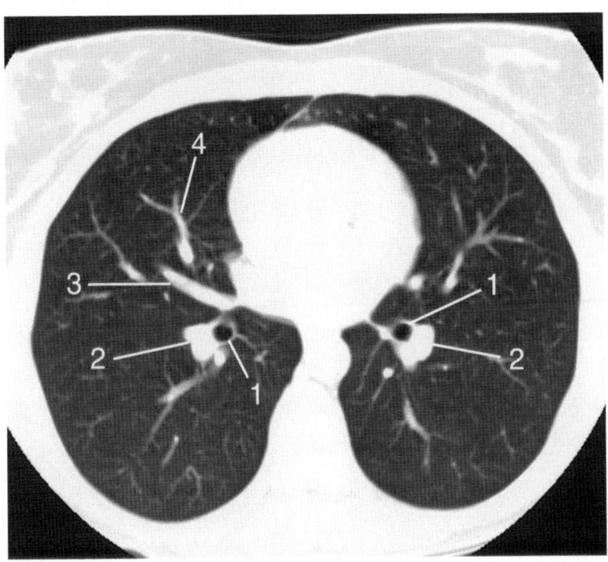

Same level as facing page.

scan level
(See image on page 51.)

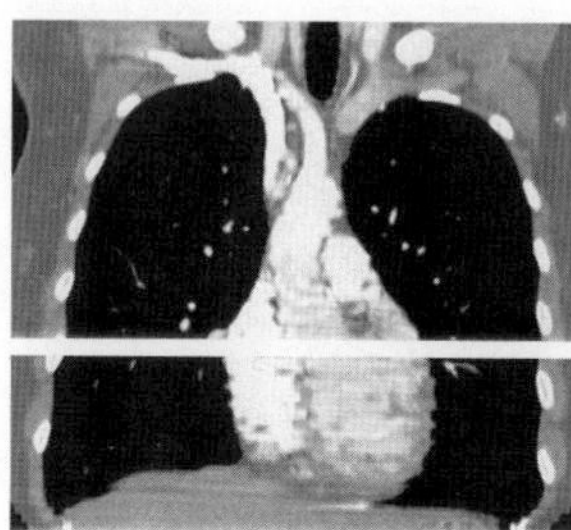

Mediastinal Window

1. ascending aorta
2. descending aorta
3. right ventricle
4. right atrium
5. left atrium
6. left atrial appendage
7. inferior pulm vein
8. segmental lower lobe art
9. left ant descending coronary art
10. circumflex coronary art

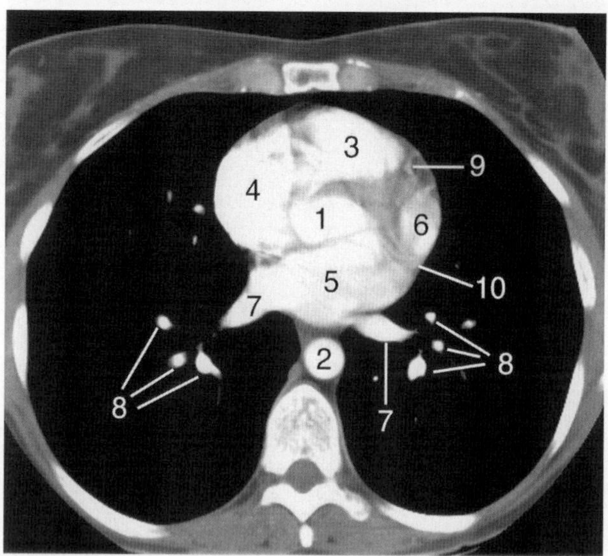

Same level as facing page.

scan level
(See image on page 50.)

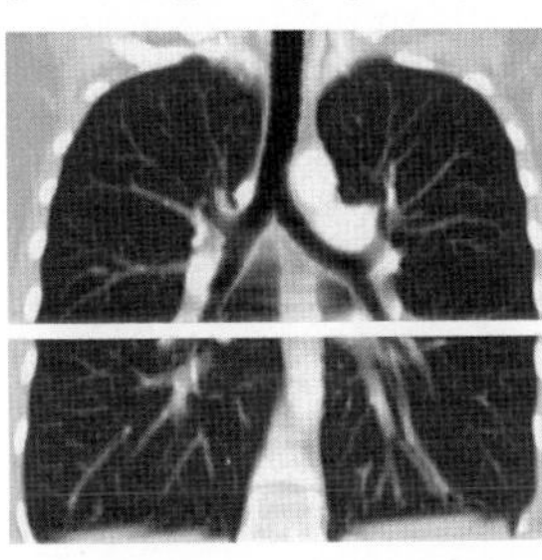

Lung Window

1. inferior pulm vein
2. anteromedial seg LLL bronchus
3. lateral seg LLL bronchus
4. post seg LLL bronchus
5. post seg RLL bronchus
6. lateral seg RLL bronchus
7. ant seg RLL bronchus
8. segmental pulm art

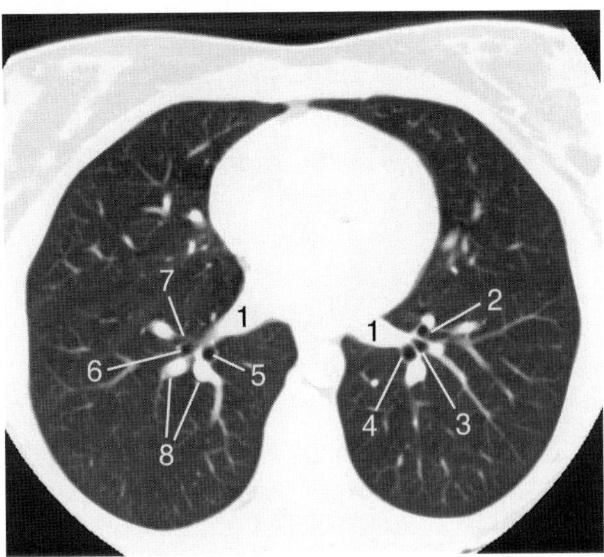

Same level as facing page.

scan level
(See image on page 51.)

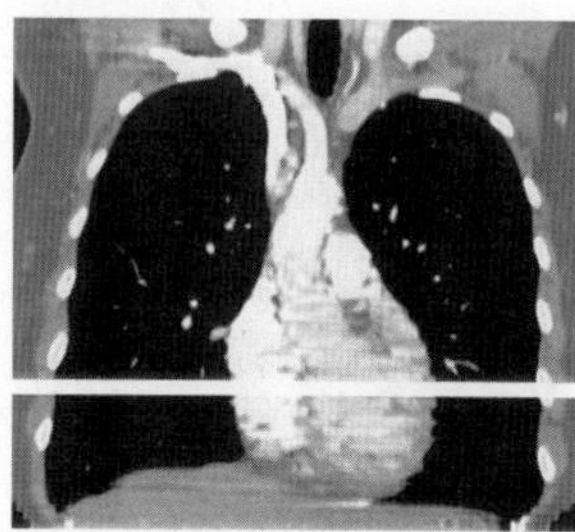

Mediastinal Window

1. left ventricle
2. left atrium
3. right atrium
4. right ventricle
5. mitral valve
6. ventricular septum

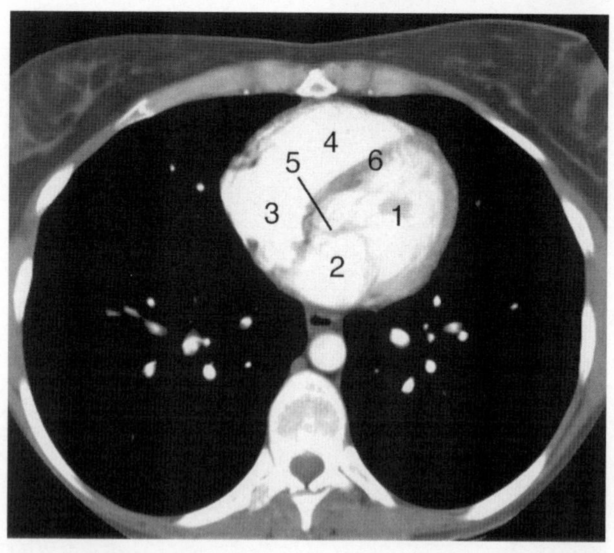

scan level
(See image on page 51.)

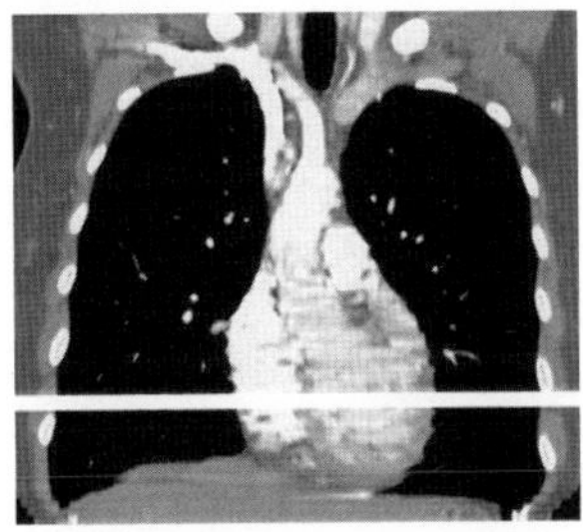

Mediastinal Window

1. left ventricle
2. papillary muscle
3. right ventricle
4. ventricular septum
5. azygos vein
6. hemiazygos vein
7. esophagus

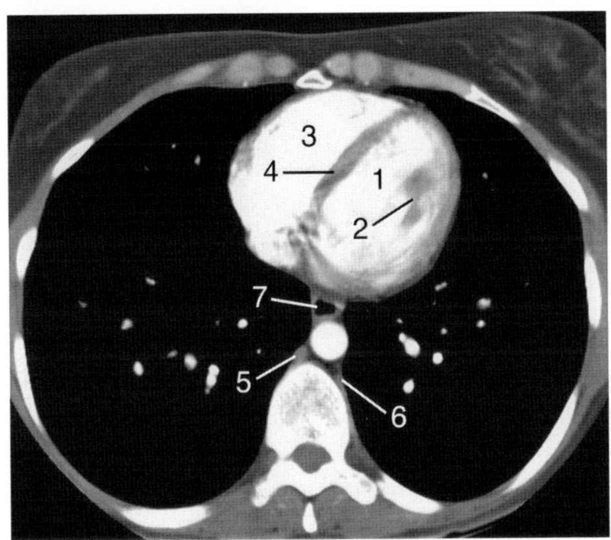

scan level
(See image on page 51.)

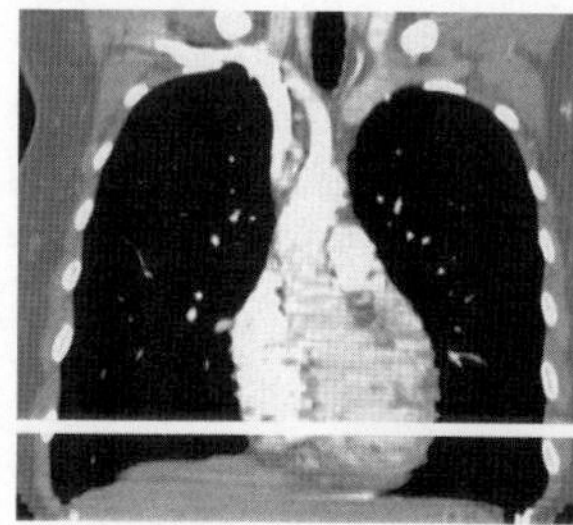

Mediastinal Window

1. left ventricle
2. right ventricle
3. inferior vena cava
4. descending aorta
5. azygos vein
6. hemiazygos vein

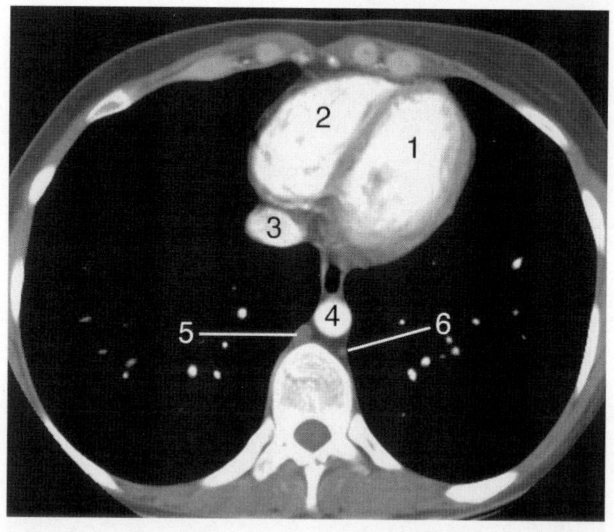

scan level
(See image on page 51.)

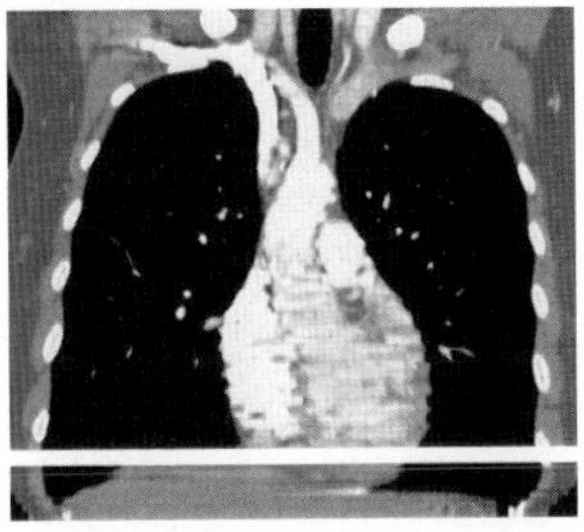

Mediastinal Window

1. apex left ventricle
2. right ventricle
3. inferior vena cava
4. liver
5. descending aorta
6. esophagus
7. azygos vein
8. hemiazygos vein
9. vertebral body
10. spinal cord

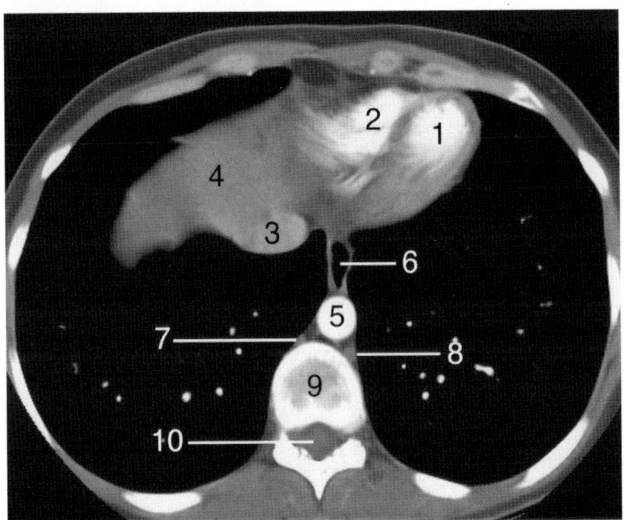

1. trachea
2. apical seg RUL bronchus
3. post seg RUL bronchus
4. apical-posterior seg LUL bronchus
5. major fissure
6. LUL
7. superior seg LLL

scan level
(See image on page 50.)

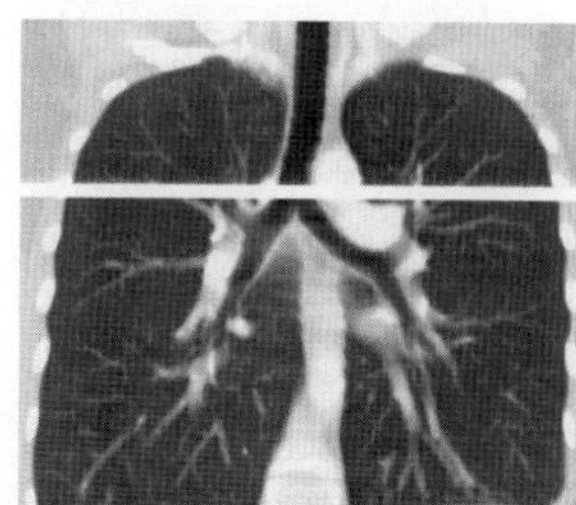

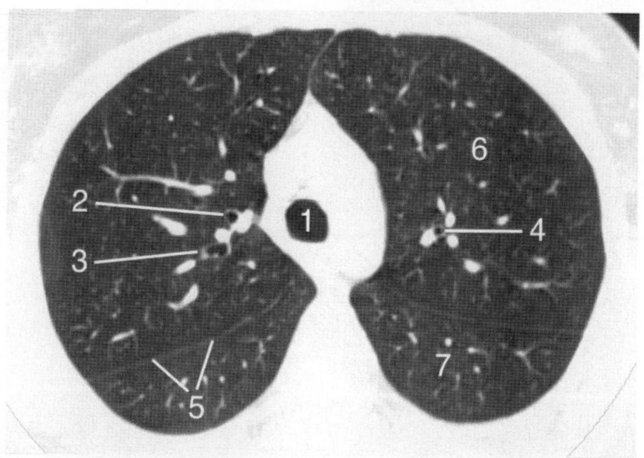

See image on page 25.

scan level
(see image on page 50.)

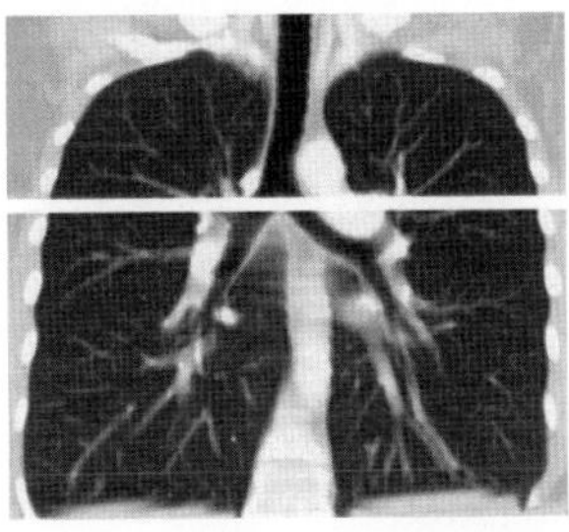

1. right main bronchus
2. left main bronchus
3. RUL bronchus
4. ant seg RUL bronchus
5. ant seg art
6. truncus ant (RUL art)
7. apical-posterior seg LUL bronchus
8. ant seg LUL art
9. major fissure
10. minor fissure

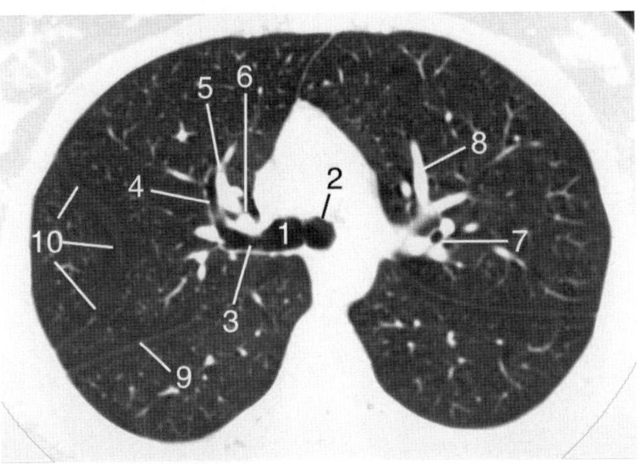

See image on page 27.

1. interlobar pulm art
2. bronchus intermedius
3. left main bronchus
4. LUL bronchus

scan level
(See image on page 50.)

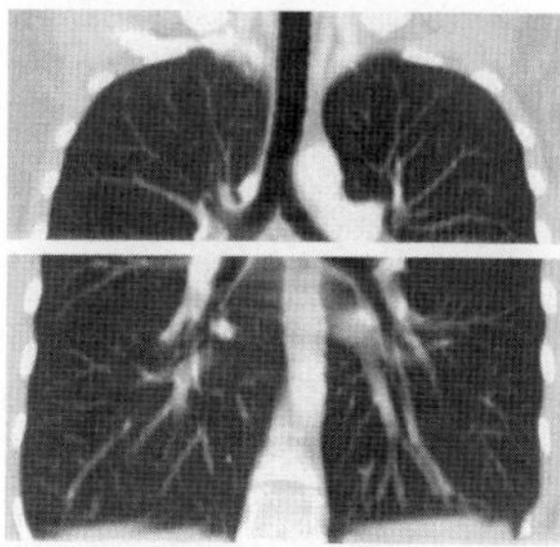

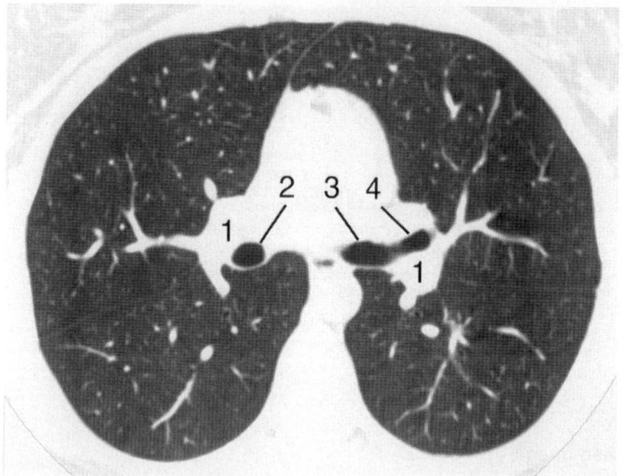

See image on page 31.

scan level
(See image on page 50.)

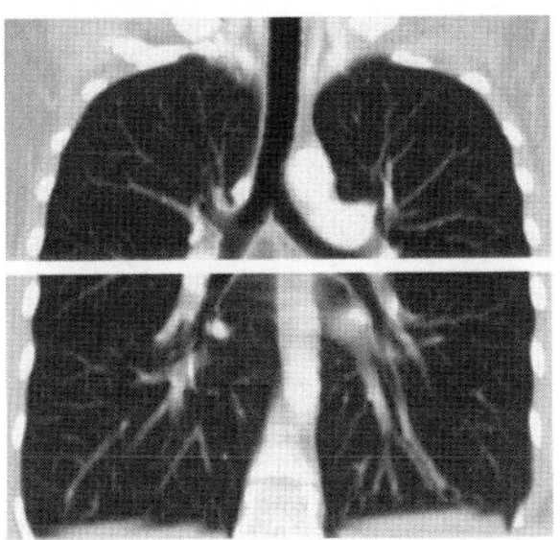

1. bronchus intermedius
2. LUL bronchus
3. lingular bronchus
4. superior lingular seg bronchus
5. superior seg lower lobe bronchus

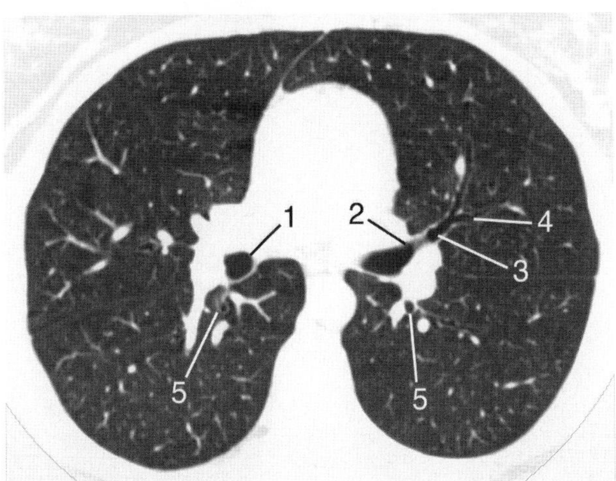

See image on page 33.

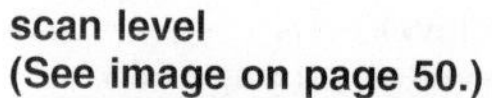

scan level
(See image on page 50.)

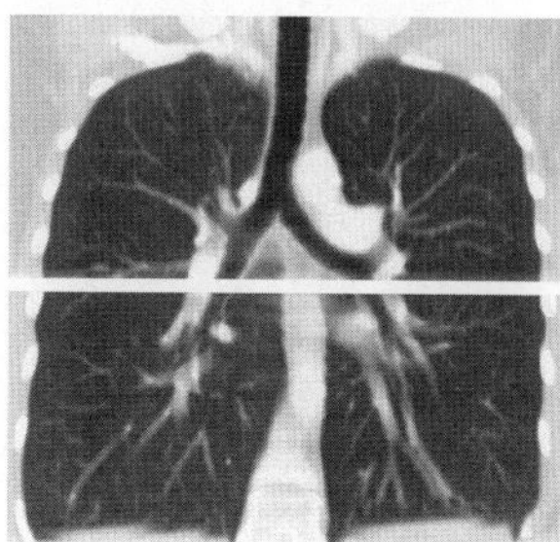

1. lower lobe pulm art
2. RML bronchus
3. lower lobe bronchus
4. superior seg lower lobe bronchus
5. superior seg lower lobe art
6. medial seg RML bronchus
7. medial seg RML art
8. lateral seg RML bronchus
9. lateral seg RML art
10. inferior seg lingula bronchus
11. inferior seg lingula art
12. lingular vein

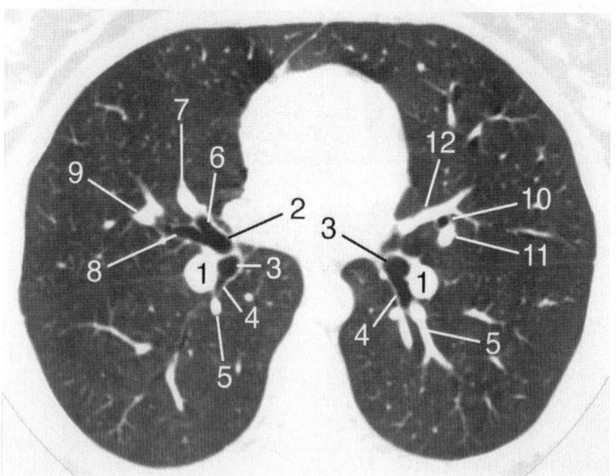

See image on page 35.

scan level
(See image on page 50.)

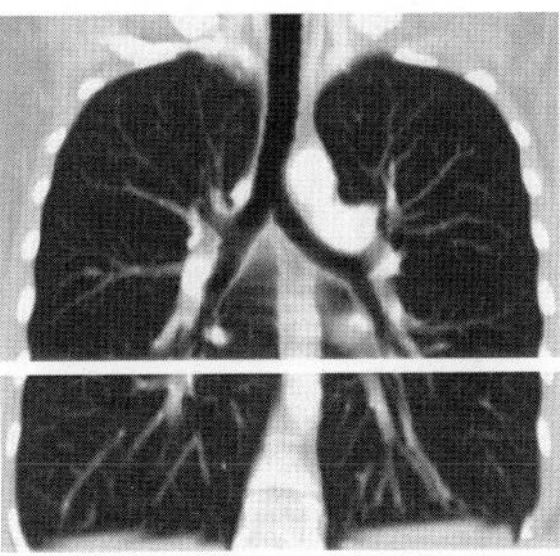

1. medial seg RLL bronchus
2. ant seg RLL bronchus
3. lateral seg RLL bronchus
4. post seg RLL bronchus
5. anteromedial seg LLL bronchus
6. lateral seg LLL bronchus
7. post seg LLL bronchus
8. inferior pulm ligament

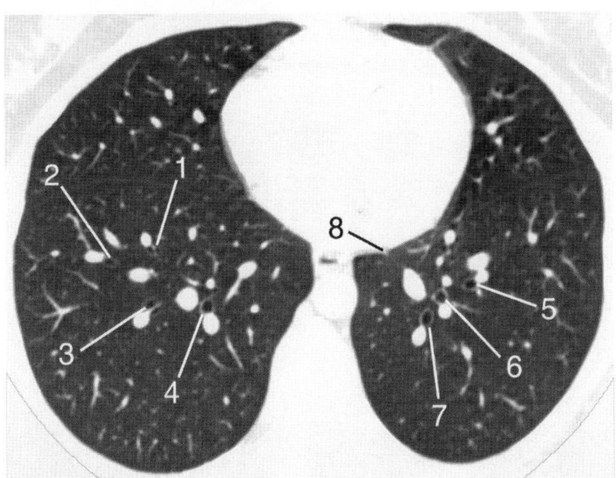

See image on page 40.

scan level
(See image on page 57.)

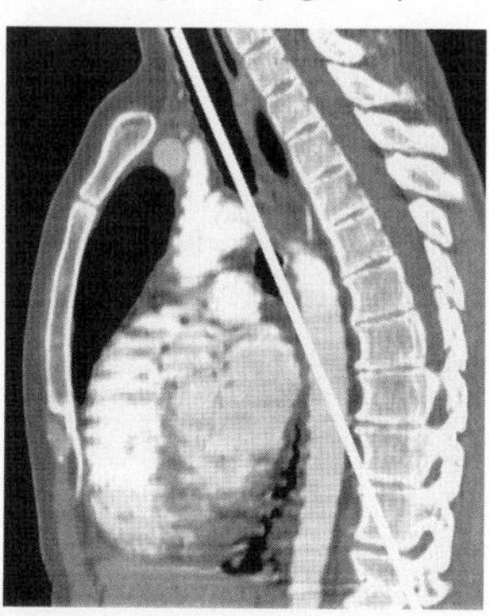

Lung Window

1. aortic arch
2. left pulm art
3. arch of azygos vein
4. interlobar pulm art
5. RUL bronchus
6. apical seg RUL bronchus
7. bronchus intermedius
8. basal seg RLL bronchi
9. inferior pulm vein
10. basal seg LLL bronchi
11. basal trunk LLL bronchus
12. LUL bronchus
13. apical-posterior seg LUL bronchus

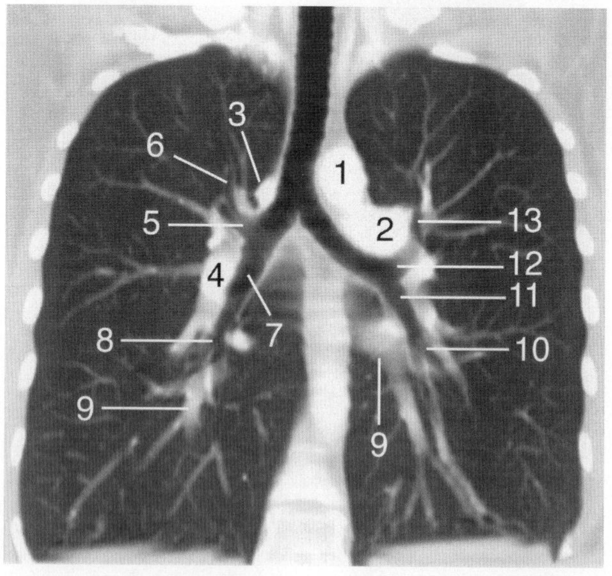

scan level
(See image on page 30.)

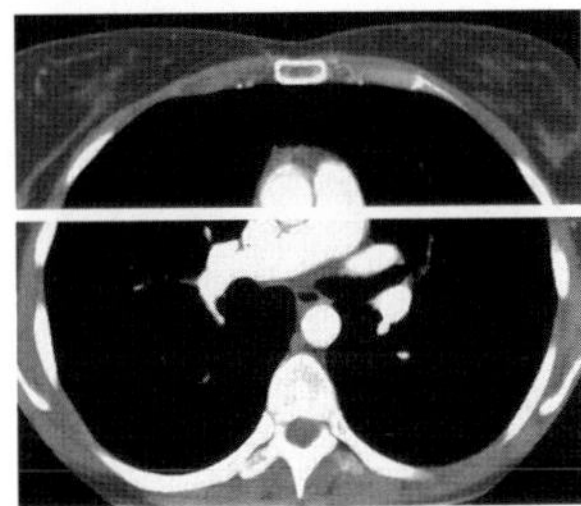

Mediastinal Window

1. right atrium
2. ascending aorta
3. aortic root
4. left ventricle
5. main pulm art
6. left atrial appendage
7. superior vena cava
8. brachiocephalic vein
9. internal jugular vein
10. trachea
11. innominate art
12. subclavian vein
13. clavicular head

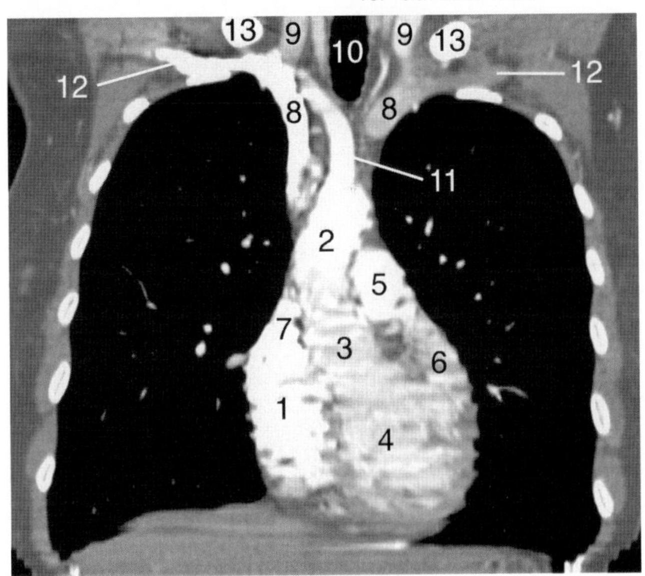

scan level
(See image on page 30.)

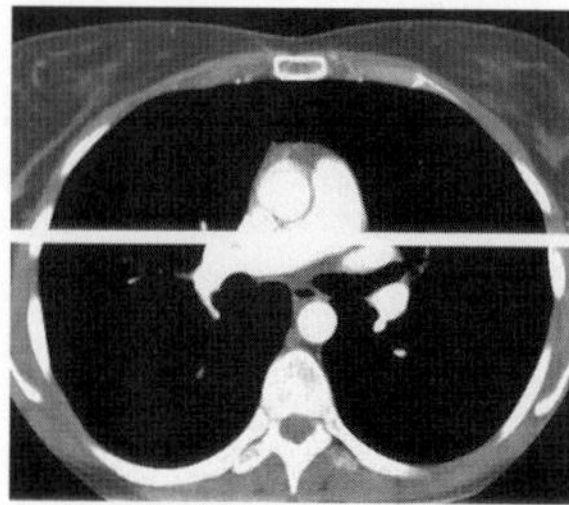

Mediastinal Window

1. left atrium
2. aortic arch
3. right pulm art
4. superior vena cava
5. superior pulm vein
6. trachea
7. esophagus
8. subclavian vein
9. subclavian art
10. vertebral art

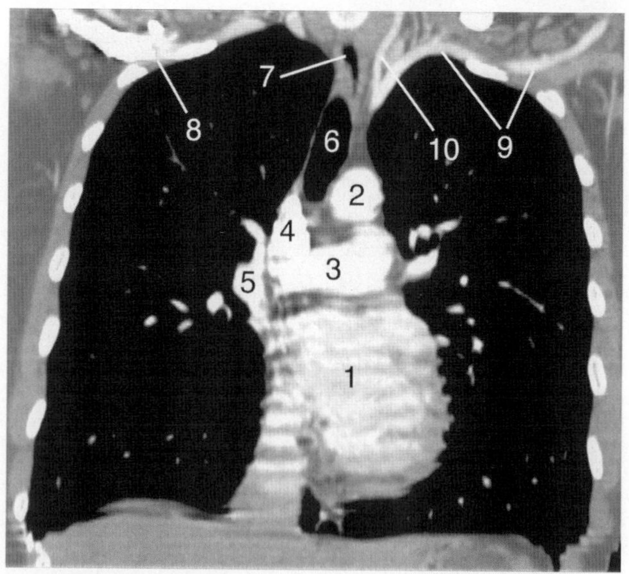

scan level
(See image on page 30.)

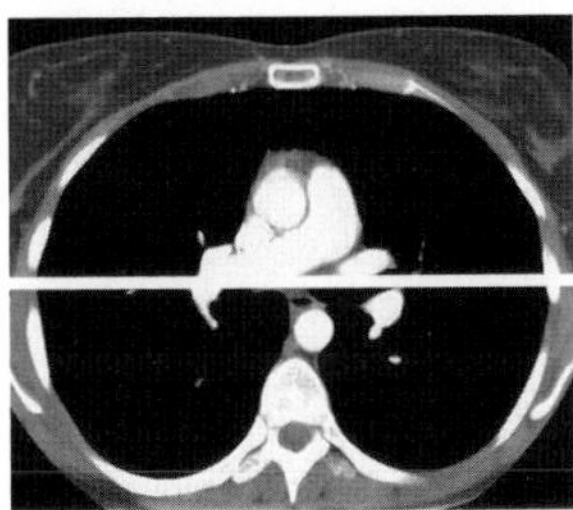

Mediastinal Window

1. aortic arch
2. left pulm art
3. right pulm art
4. left atrium
5. tracheal carina
6. truncus ant
7. right superior pulm vein
8. interlobar pulm art
9. left superior pulm vein
10. subclavian art
11. esophagus

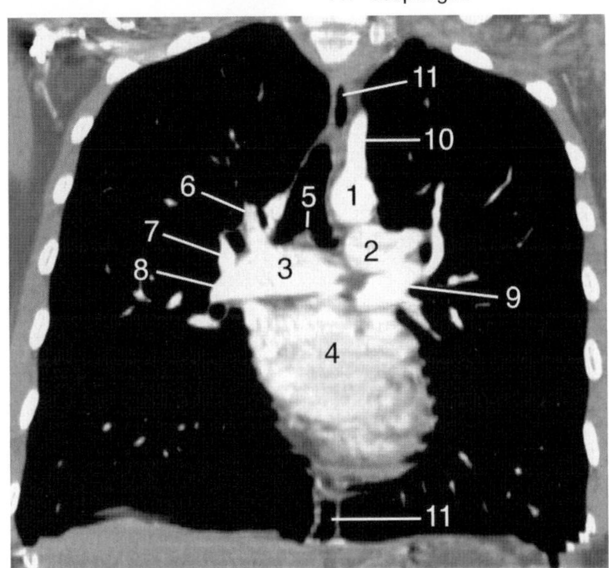

scan level
(See image on page 30.)

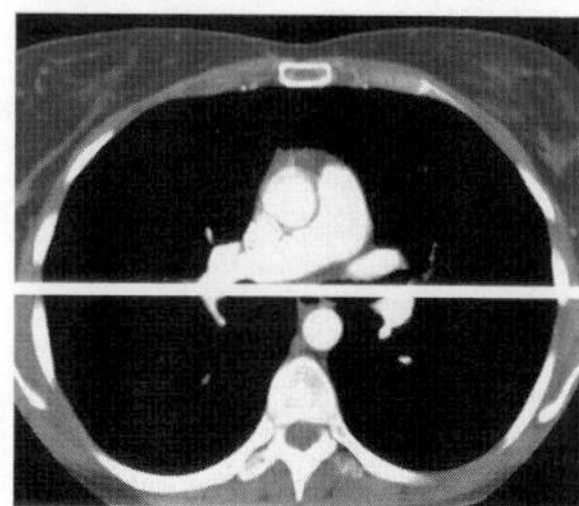

Mediastinal Window

1. right main bronchus
2. left main bronchus
3. aortic arch
4. left pulm art
5. interlobar pulm art
6. left atrium
7. subcarinal space
8. RUL bronchus
9. LUL bronchus
10. esophagus
11. vertebral body

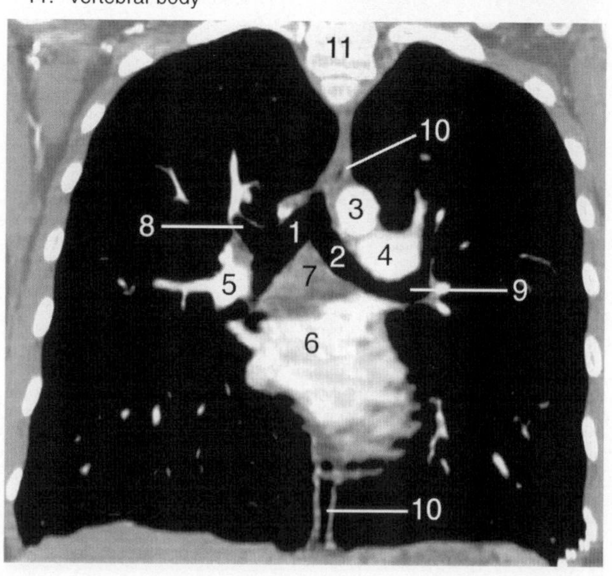

scan level
(See image on page 30.)

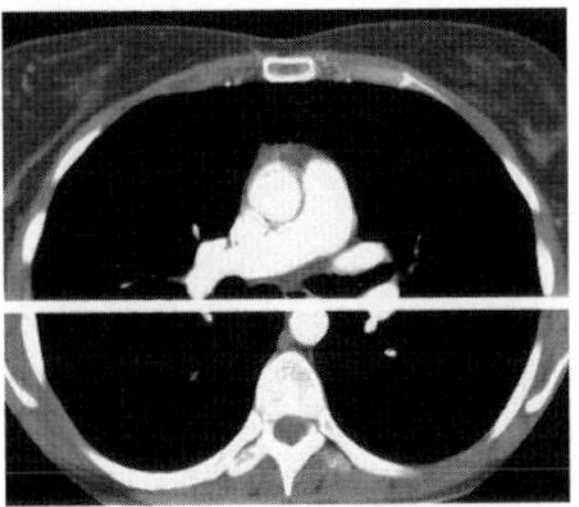

Mediastinal Window

1. descending aorta
2. interlobar pulm art
3. bronchus intermedius
4. basal trunk LLL bronchus
5. inferior pulm vein

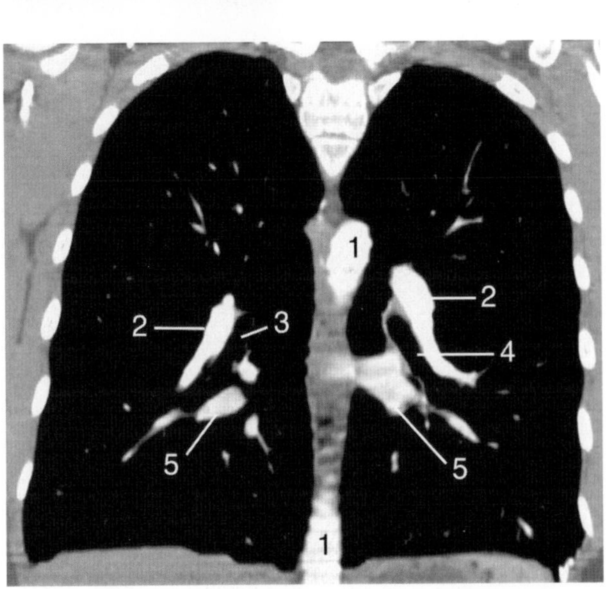

scan level
(See image on page 30.)

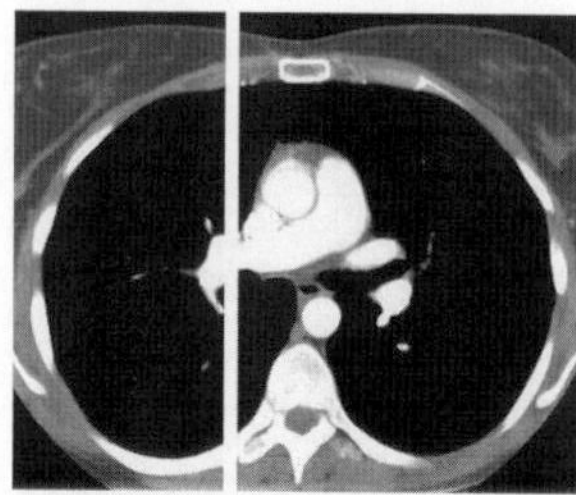

Mediastinal Window

1. right interlobar pulm art
2. truncus ant (RUL art)
3. right superior pulm vein
4. RUL bronchus
5. bronchus intermedius
6. right inferior pulm vein
7. right subclavian vein
8. right subclavian art
9. clavicle
10. right atrium
11. inferior vena cava

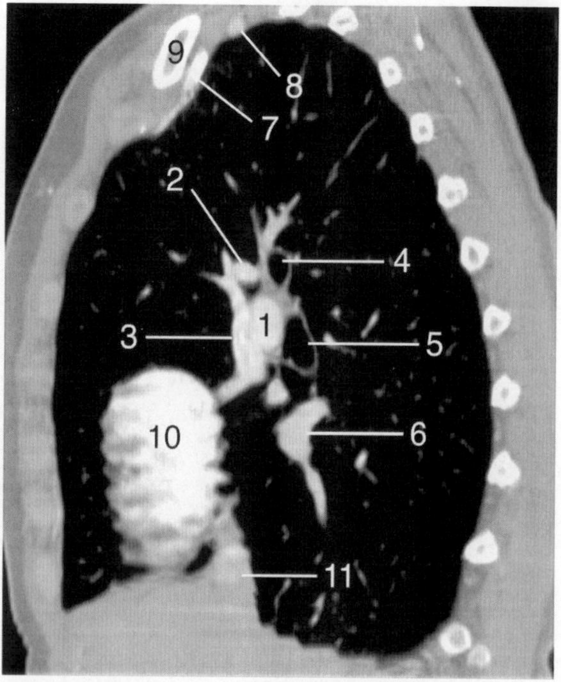

scan level
(See image on page 30.)

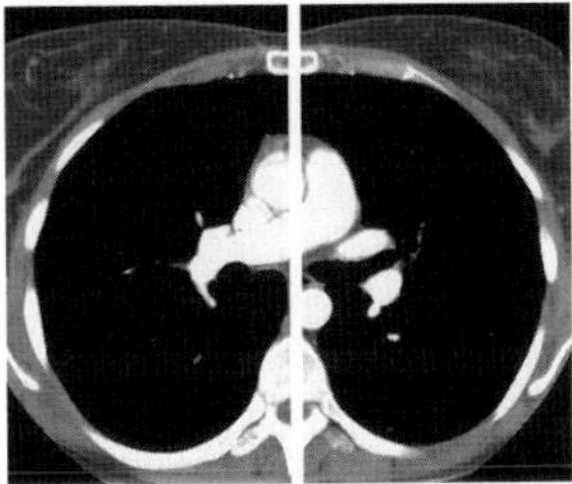

Mediastinal Window

1. aortic arch
2. descending aorta
3. innominate art
4. left brachiocephalic vein
5. right pulm art
6. right ventricle
7. left atrium
8. trachea
9. esophagus
10. spinal cord

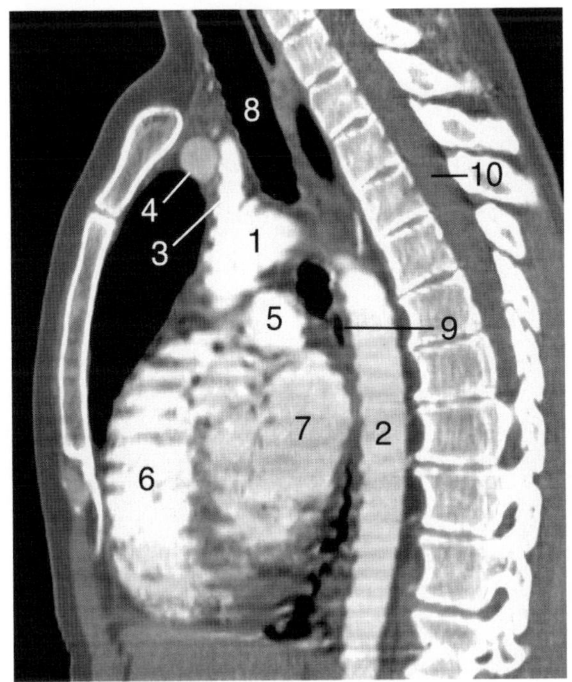

scan level
(See image on page 30.)

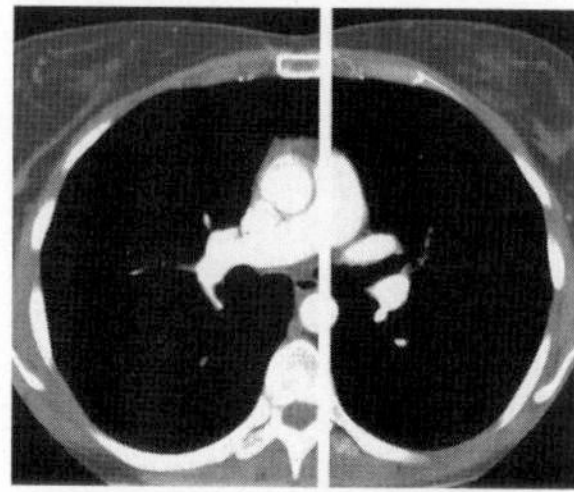

Mediastinal Window

1. aortic arch
2. left subclavian art
3. left carotid art
4. left brachiocephalic vein
5. manubrium
6. left main bronchus
7. main pulm art
8. right ventricle
9. left atrium

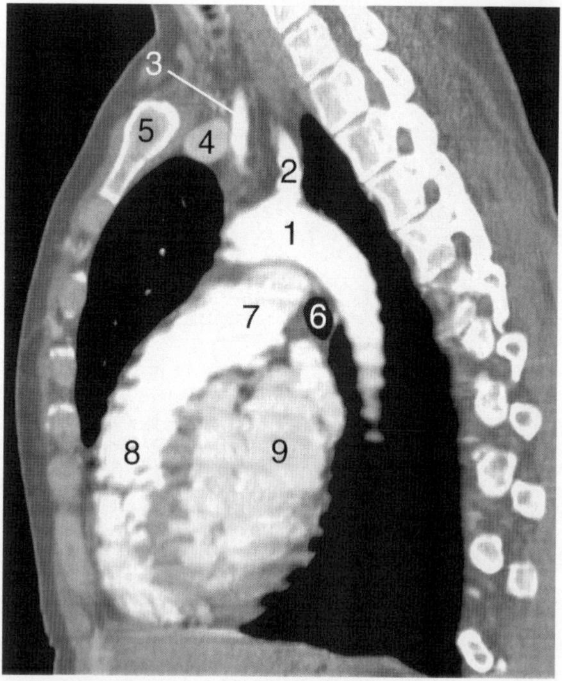

scan level
(See image on page 30.)

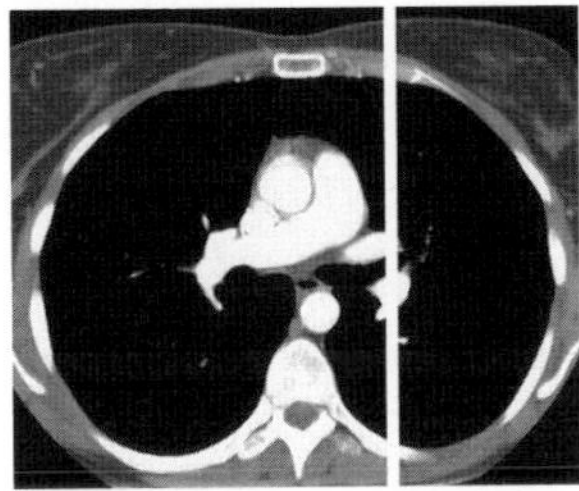

Mediastinal Window

1. interlobar left pulm art
2. LUL bronchus
3. ant seg LUL bronchus
4. apical-posterior seg LUL bronchus
5. segmental LLL bronchi
6. left inferior pulm vein
7. left ventricle
8. left superior pulm vein
9. left subclavian art
10. clavicle

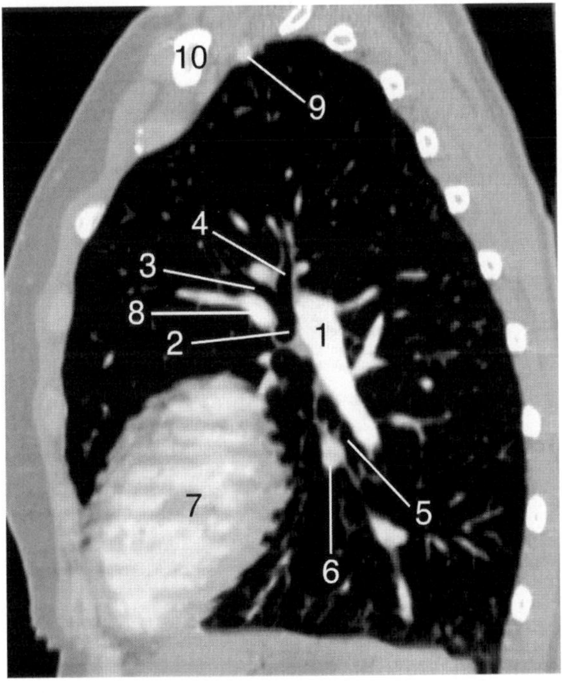

Abdomen, Portal Venous Phase

Abdomen, Portal Venous Phase/Axial

1. left hepatic vein
2. middle hepatic vein
3. right hepatic vein
4. serratus ant muscle
5. latissimus dorsi muscle
6. azygous vein
7. hemiazygous vein
8. inferior vena cava
9. erector spinae muscles

A, abdominal aorta
Stom, stomach

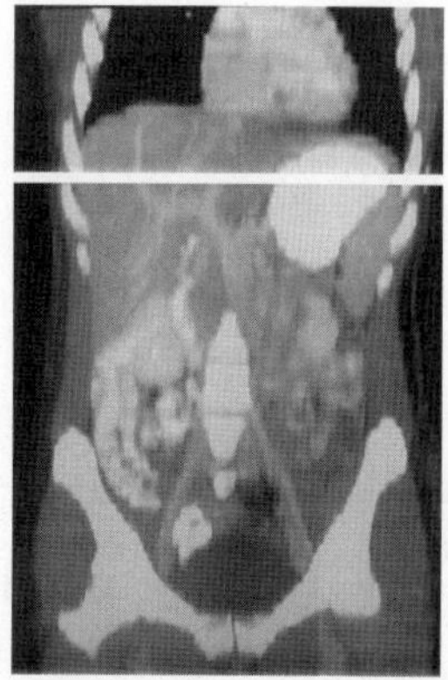

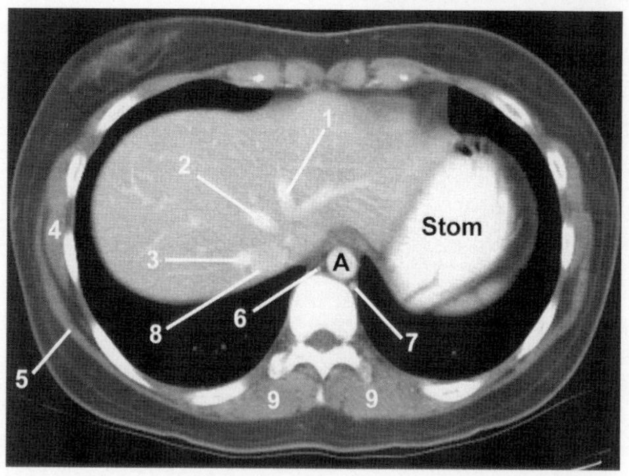

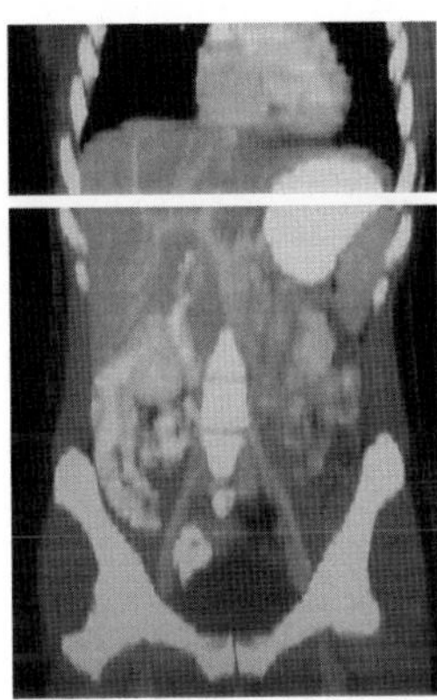

1. left hepatic vein
2. middle hepatic vein
3. right hepatic vein
4. hemiazygous vein
5. inferior vena cava
6. gastroesophageal junction

A, abdominal aorta
Spl, spleen
Stom, stomach

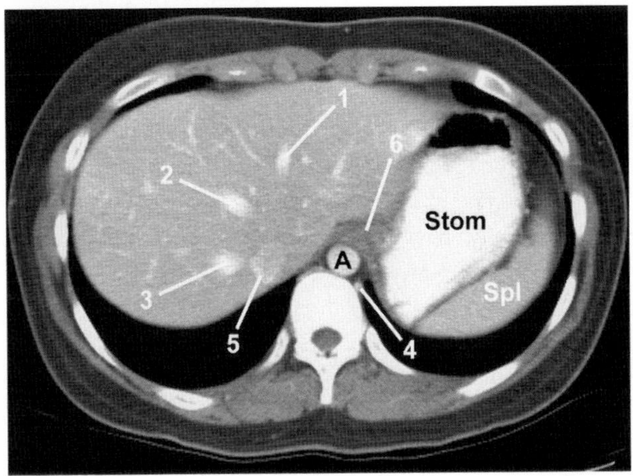

1. middle hepatic vein
2. inferior vena cava

AS, ant seg right lobe of liver
LS, lateral seg left lobe of liver
MS, medial seg left lobe of liver
PS, post seg right lobe of liver
Spl, spleen
Stom, stomach

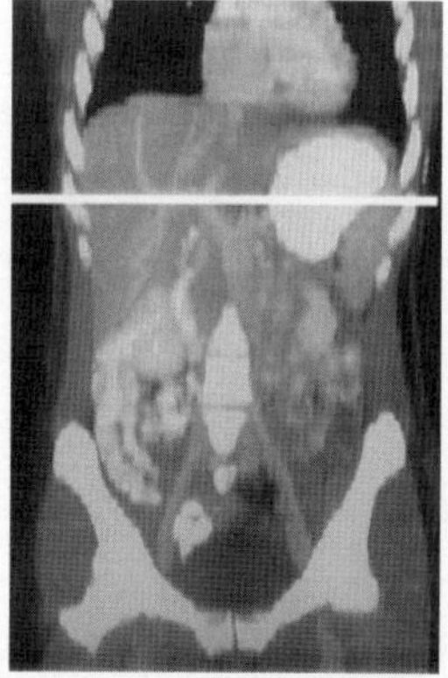

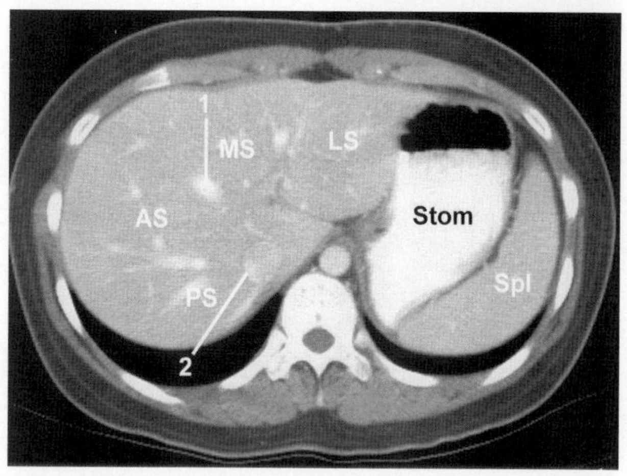

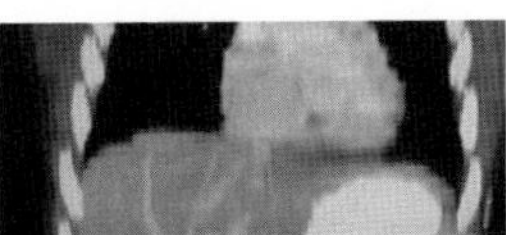

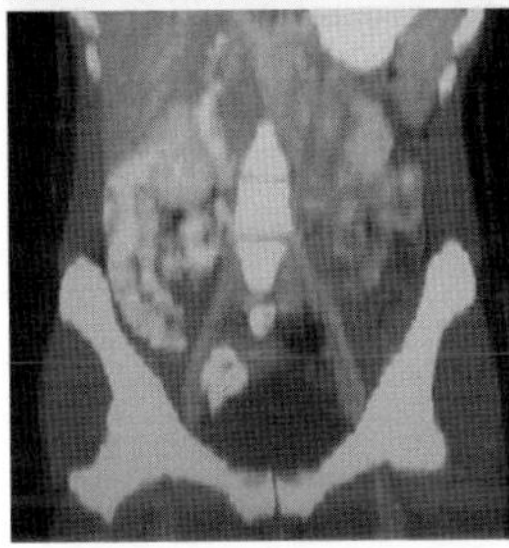

1. middle hepatic vein
2. left portal vein
3. inferior vena cava

AS, ant seg left lobe of liver
LS, lateral seg left lobe of liver
MS, medial seg left lobe of liver
PS, post seg right lobe of liver
Spl, spleen
Stom, stomach

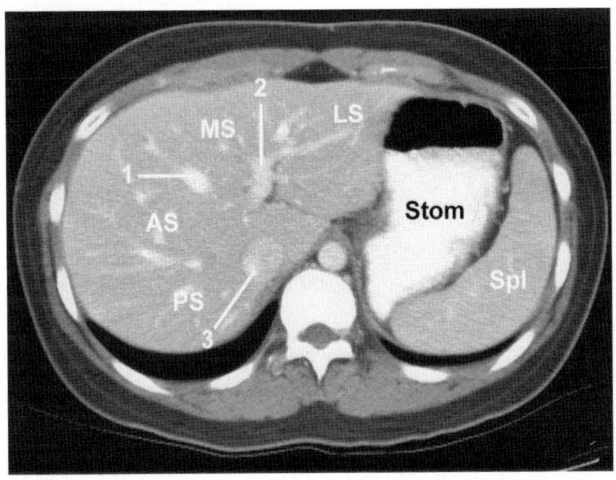

Abdomen, Portal Venous Phase/Axial

1. main portal vein
2. inferior vena cava
3. splenic vein
4. pancreas (body)

A, abdominal aorta
Spl, spleen
Stom, stomach

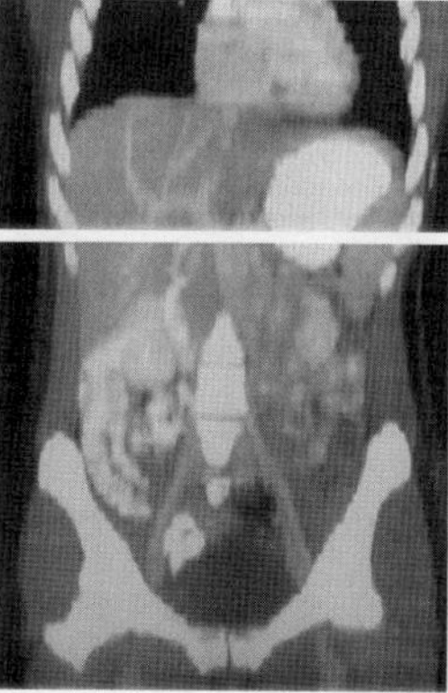

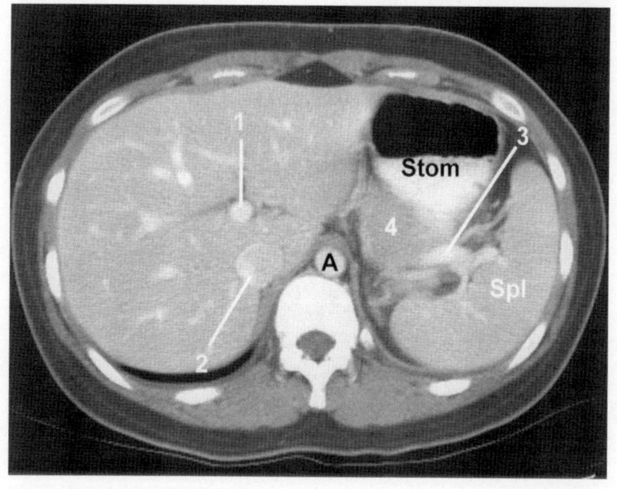

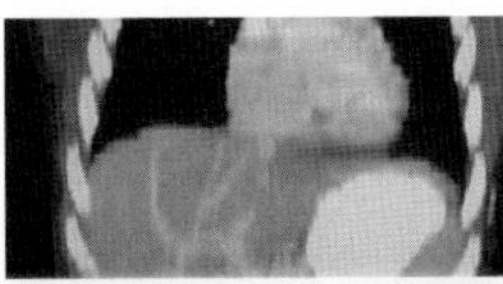
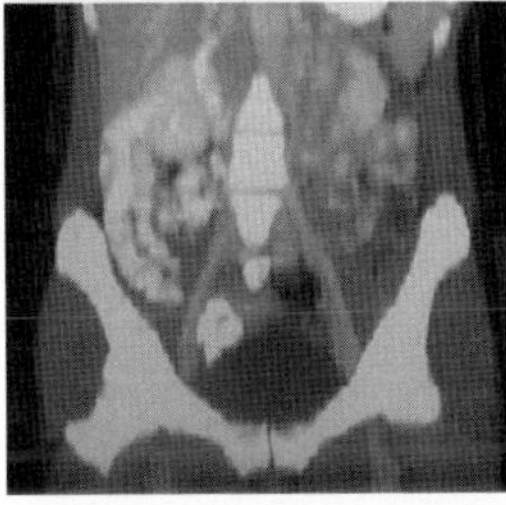

1. main portal vein
2. splenic vein
3. crus of diaphragm
4. pancreas (body)
5. caudate lobe of liver
6. hepatic art
7. inferior vena cava

LS, lateral seg left lobe of liver
MS, medial seg left lobe of liver
Spl, spleen
Stom, stomach

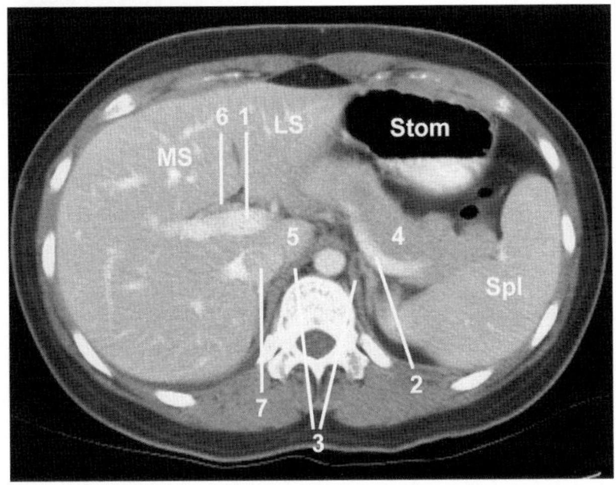

Abdomen, Portal Venous Phase/Axial

1. main portal vein
2. splenic vein
3. adrenal glands
4. pancreas
5. colon: splenic flexure
6. common bile duct
7. right portal vein

J, jejunum
Spl, spleen
Stom, stomach

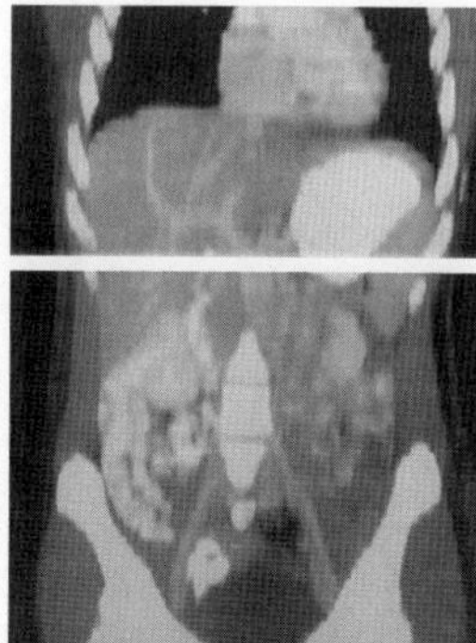

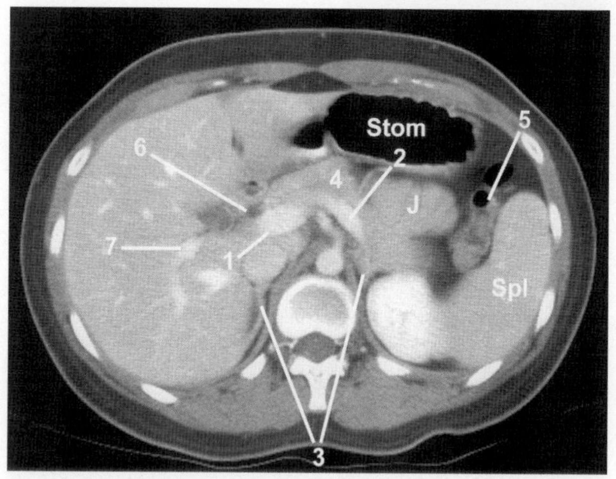

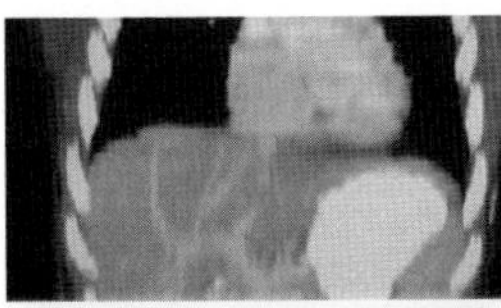

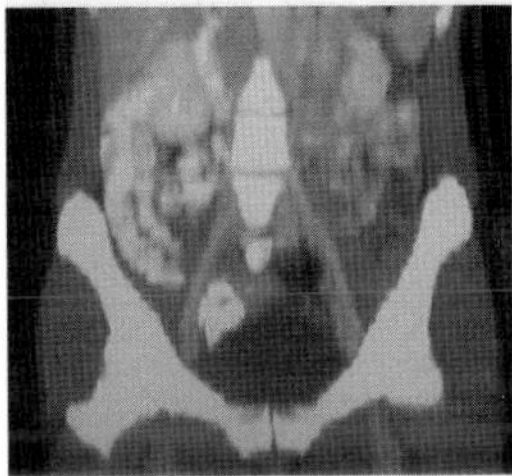

1. portosplenic vein confluence
2. splenic vein
3. vertebral body
4. pancreas (neck)
5. adrenal glands
6. colon: splenic flexure
7. right portal vein
8. common bile duct

J, jejunum
LK, left kidney
Spl, spleen
Stom, stomach

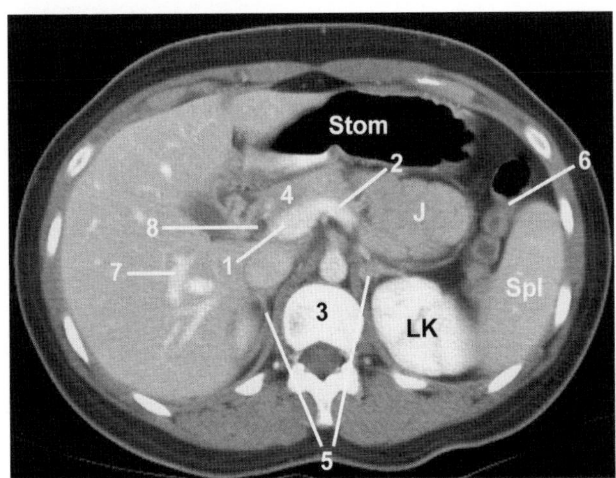

Abdomen, Portal Venous Phase/Axial

1. superior mesenteric vein
2. superior mesenteric art
3. crus of diaphragm
4. pancreas (head)
5. common bile duct
6. duodenum
7. gallbladder
8. colon: splenic flexure

A, abdominal aorta
J, jejunum
LK, left kidney
RK, right kidney
Stom, stomach

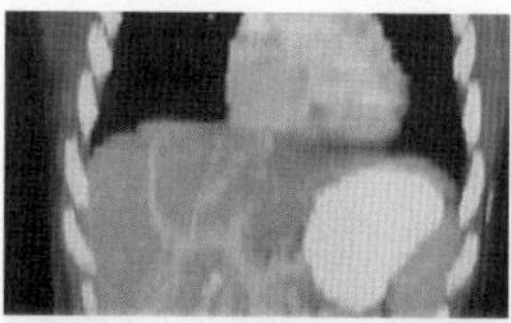

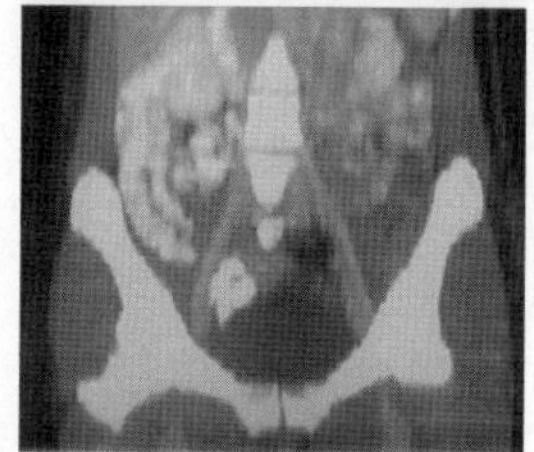

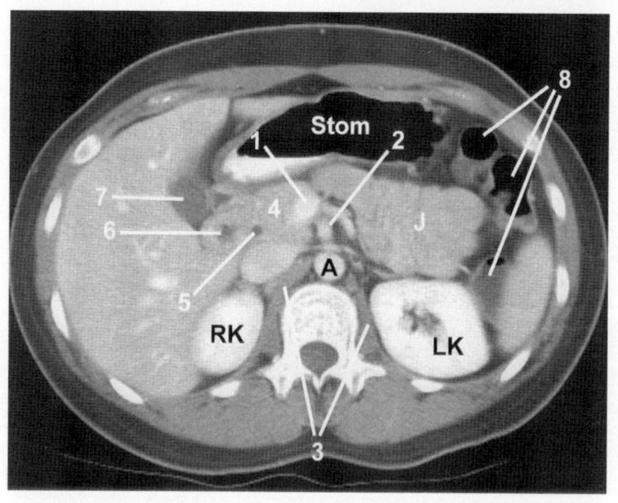

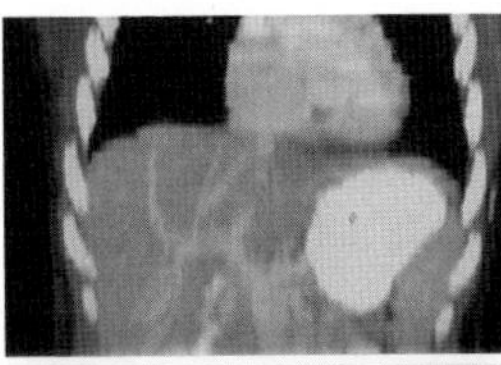

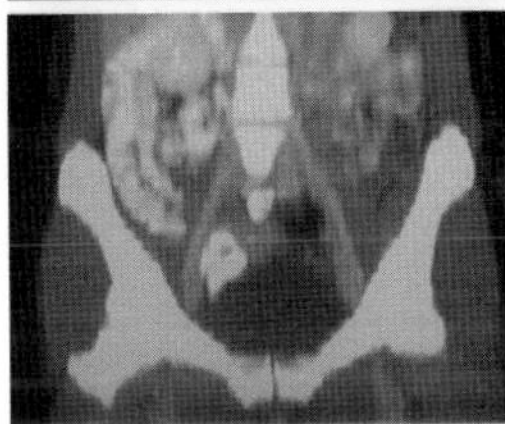

1. superior mesenteric vein
2. duodenum
3. superior mesenteric art
4. pancreas (head)
5. left renal vein
6. left renal art
7. pancreas (uncinate process)

GB, gallbladder
J, jejunum
LK, left kidney
RK, right kidney

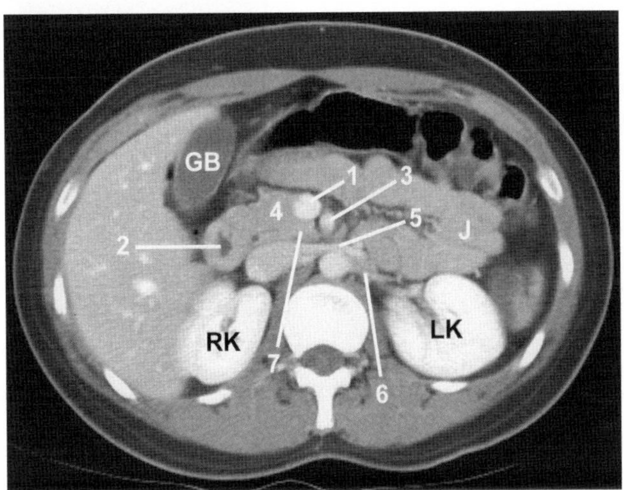

Abdomen, Portal Venous Phase/Axial

1. superior mesenteric vein
2. superior mesenteric art
3. left renal vein
4. right renal vein
5. inferior vena cava
6. pancreas
7. descending colon
8. ascending colon
9. duodenum

GB, gallbladder
J, jejunum
LK, left kidney
RK, right kidney

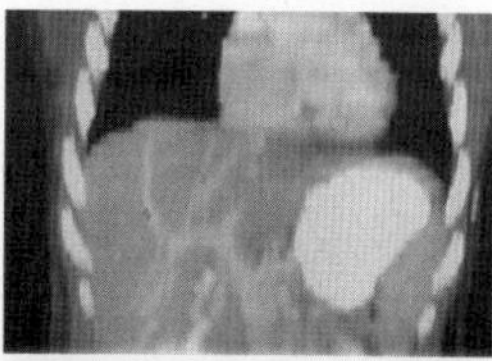

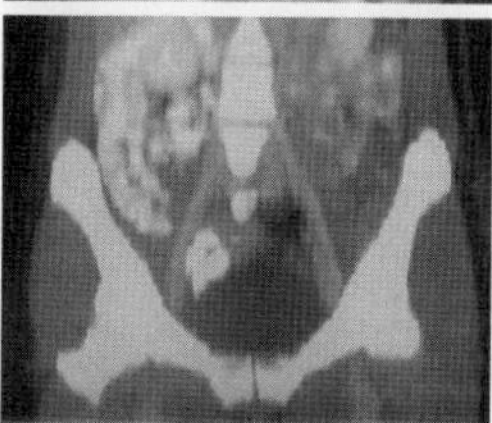

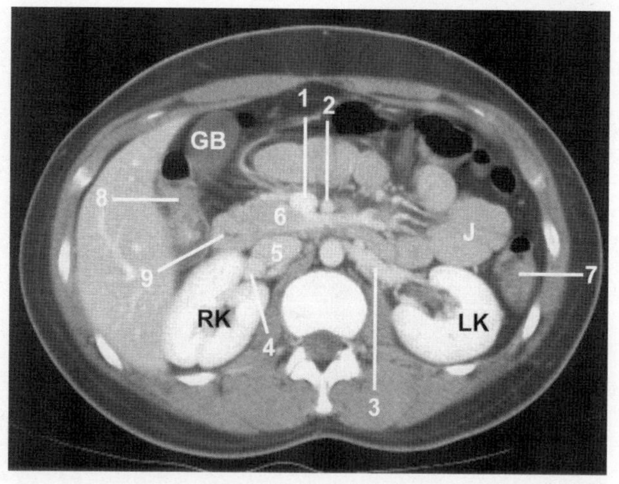

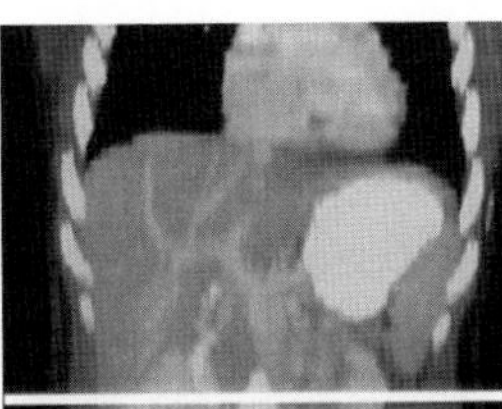
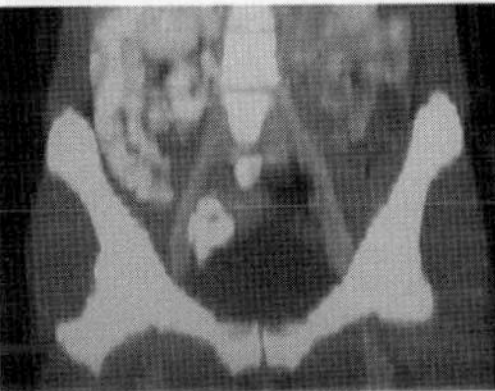

1. superior mesenteric vein
2. superior mesenteric art
3. duodenum
4. right renal art
5. descending colon

J, jejunum
L, liver
LK, left kidney
RK, right kidney

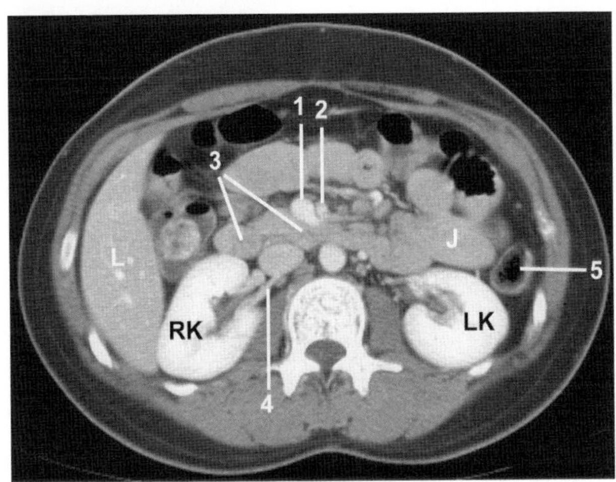

Abdomen, Portal Venous Phase/Axial

1. duodenum
2. inferior vena cava
3. right renal collecting system (renal pelvis)
4. descending colon
5. vertebral body
6. spinous process of vertebral body

A, abdominal aorta
J, jejunum
LK, left kidney
RK, right kidney

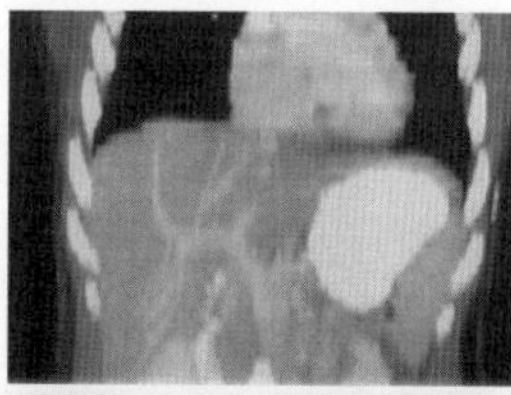

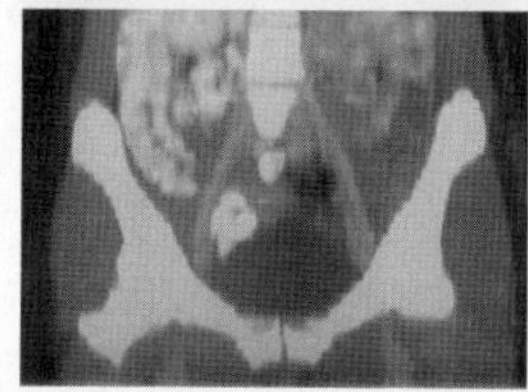

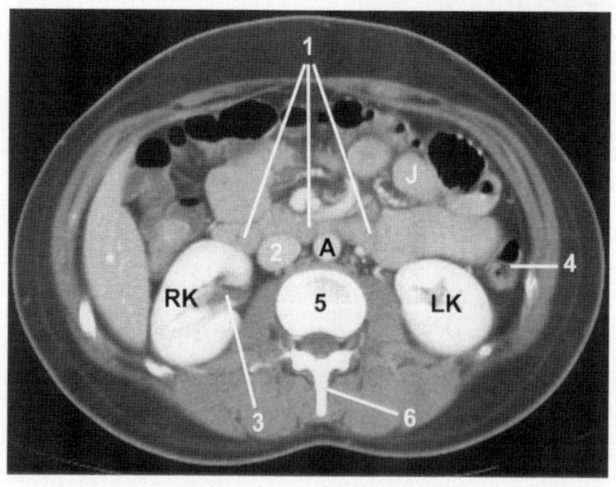

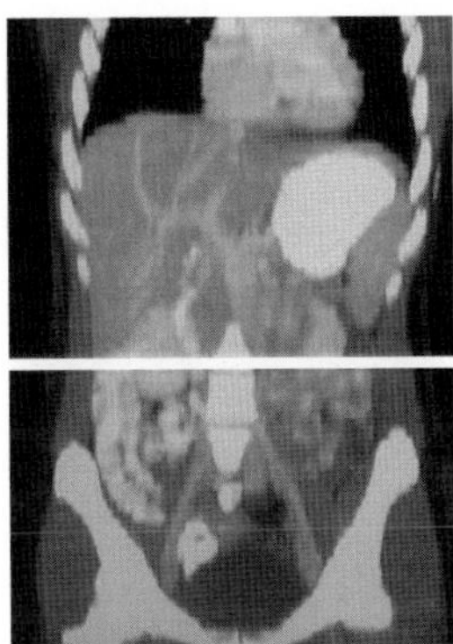

1. transverse colon
2. descending colon
3. ascending colon
4. duodenum

LK, left kidney
RK, right kidney

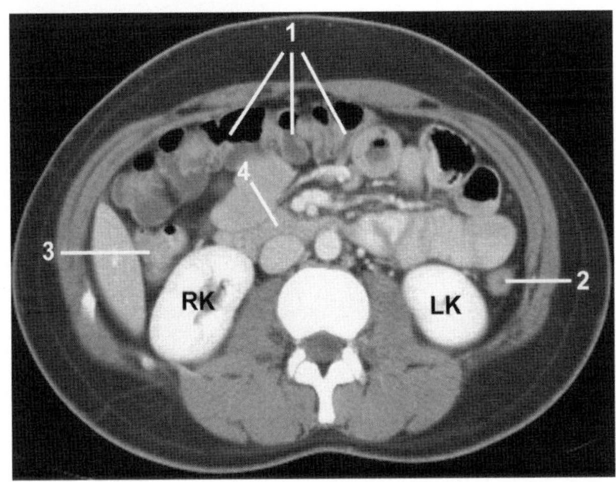

Abdomen, Portal Venous Phase/Axial

1. descending colon
2. ascending colon
3. rectus abdominus muscles
4. transversus abdominus muscle
5. internal oblique muscle
6. external oblique muscle
7. vertebral body laminae
8. vertebral body pedicles

J, jejunum
Ps, psoas muscles

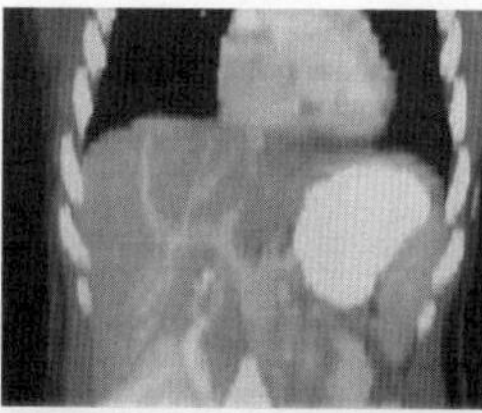

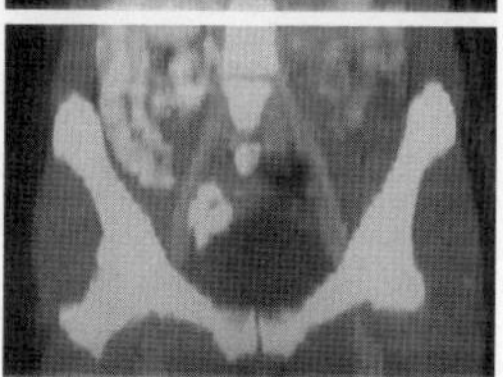

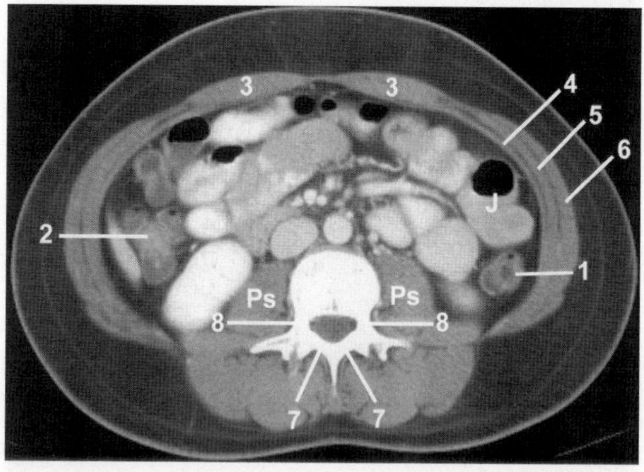

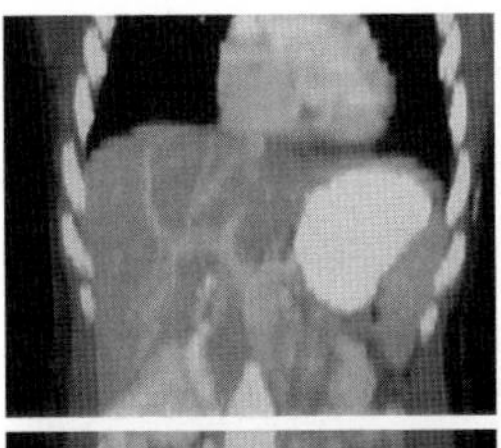

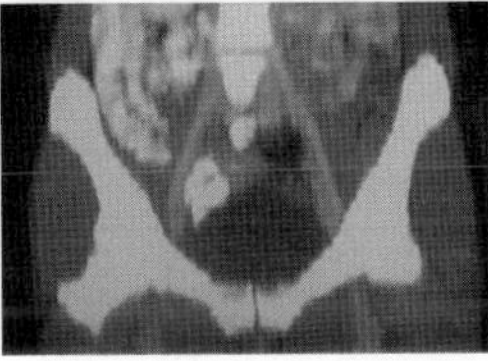

1. descending colon
2. lumbar nerve exiting neural foramen

DS, intervertebral disc space
J, jejunum
Ps, psoas muscles
QL, quadratus lumborum muscles

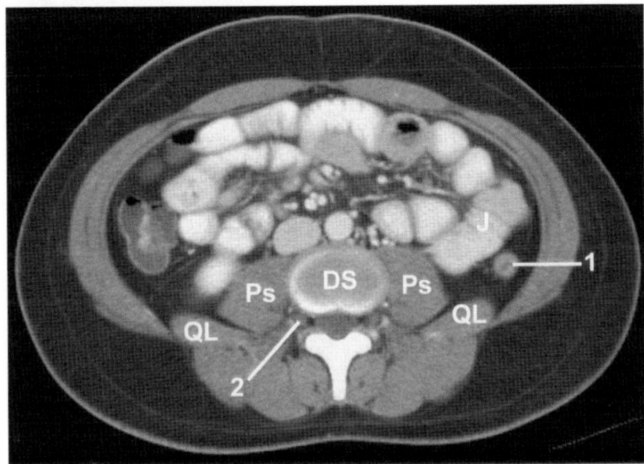

Abdomen, Portal Venous Phase/Axial

1. descending colon
2. ascending colon
3. rectus abdominus muscles

J, jejunum
Ps, psoas muscles
QL, quadratus lumborum

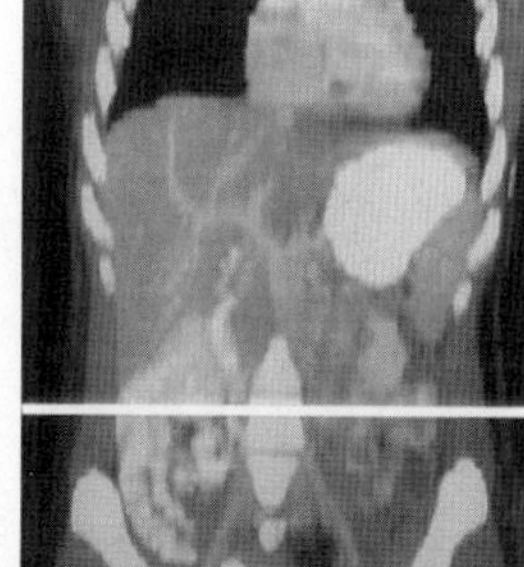

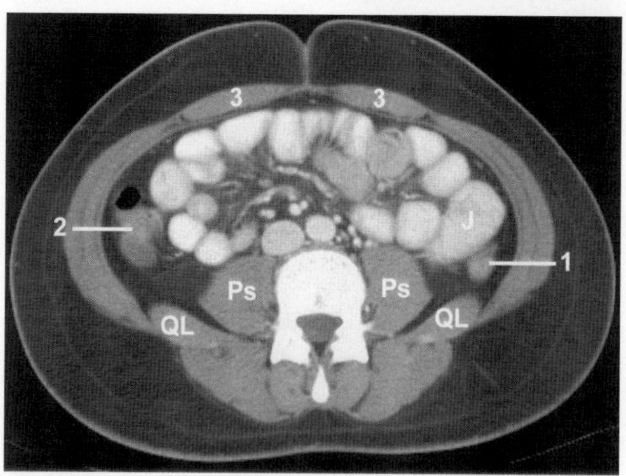

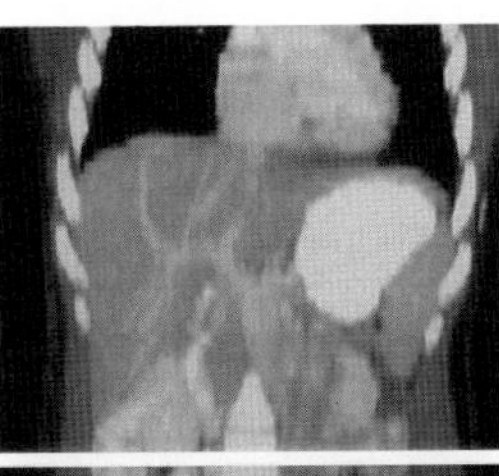

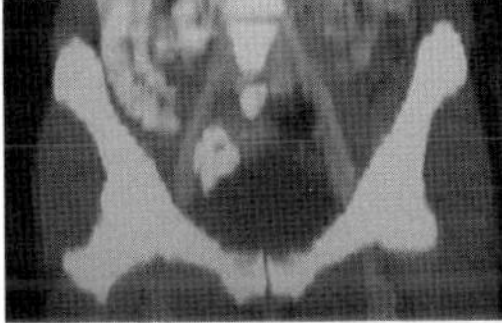

1. descending colon
2. ascending colon
3. common iliac art
4. erector spinae muscles

I, ileal bowel loops
Ps, psoas muscles

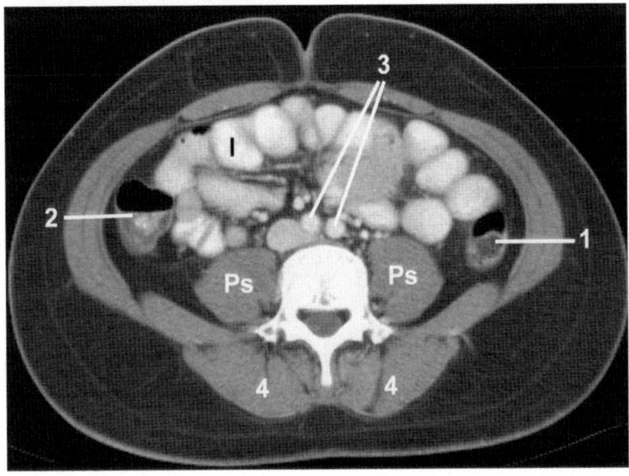

Abdomen, Portal Venous Phase/Axial

1. descending colon
2. erector spinae muscles
3. ascending colon
4. common iliac art

Ps, psoas muscles

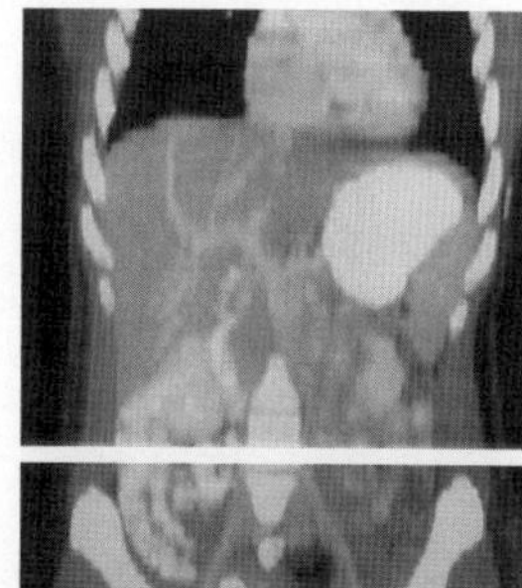

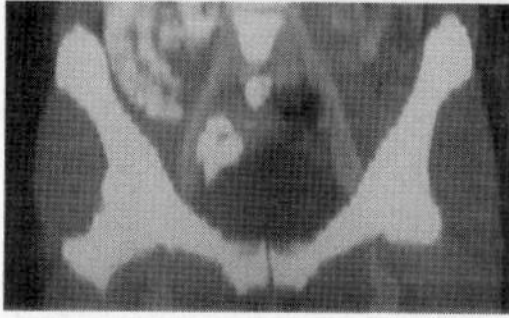

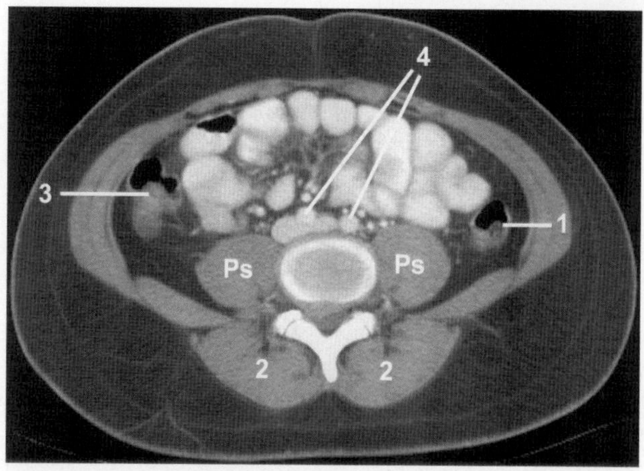

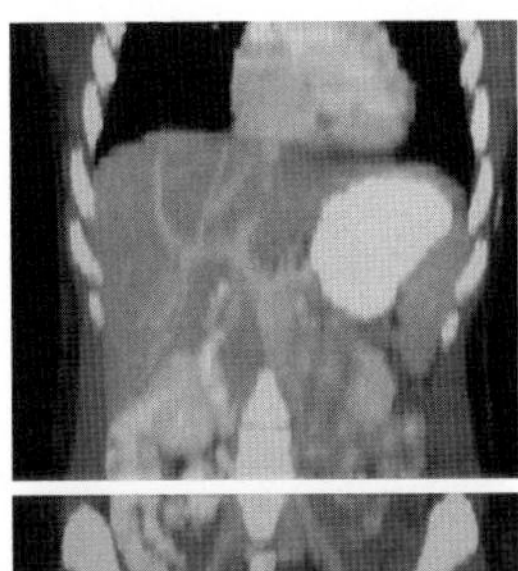

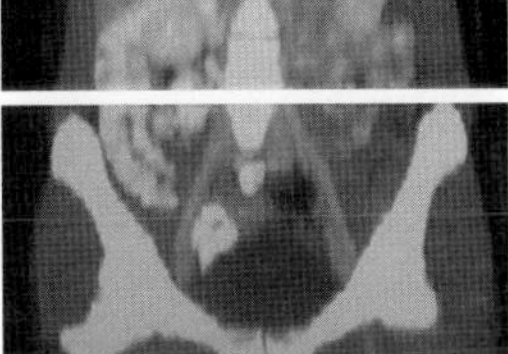

1. descending colon
2. ascending colon
3. common iliac art
4. common iliac veins

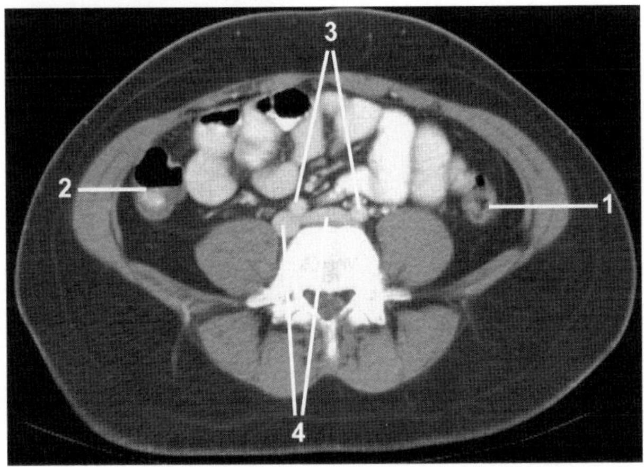

Pelvis

Portal Venous Phase

1. descending colon
2. ascending colon
3. common iliac art
4. common iliac veins
5. iliac wings

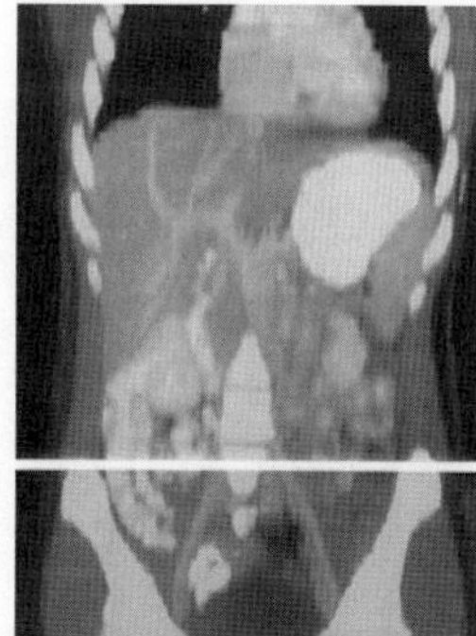

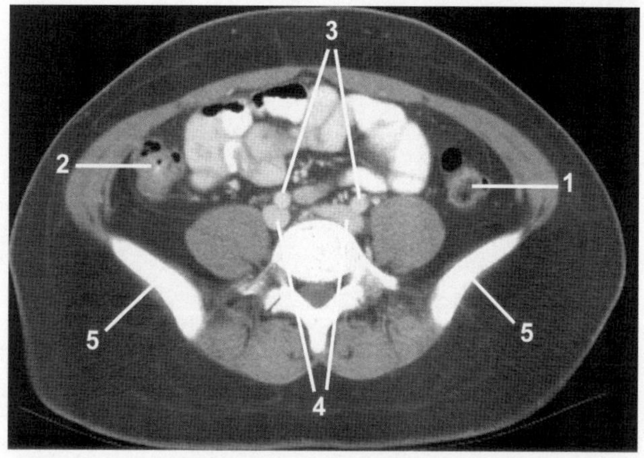

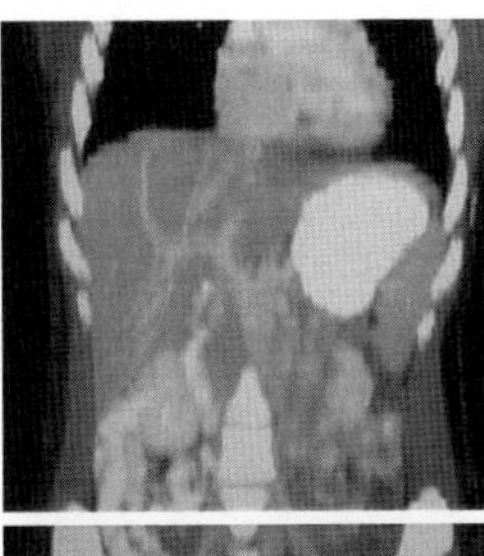

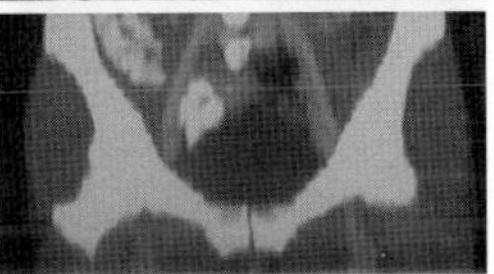

Portal Venous Phase

1. iliac wing
2. thecal sac
3. ascending colon
4. iliacus muscle
5. sacrum

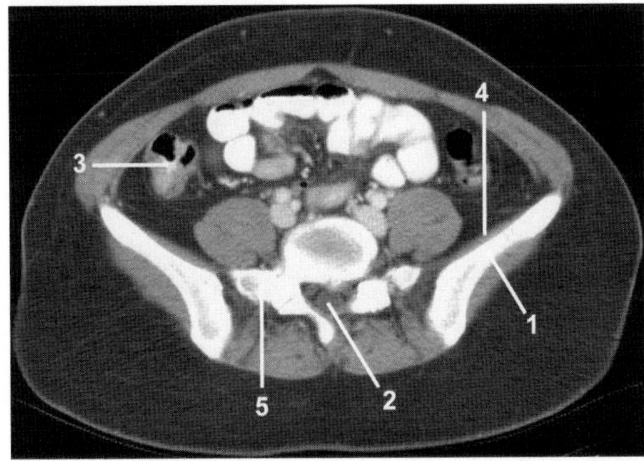

Portal Venous Phase

1. left sacroiliac joint
2. cecum
3. gluteus medius muscle

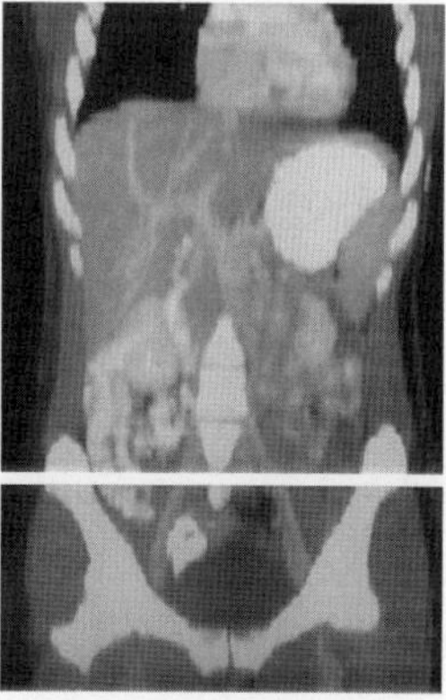

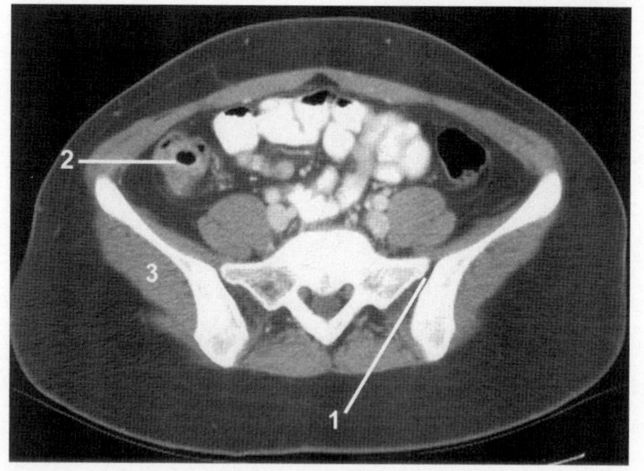

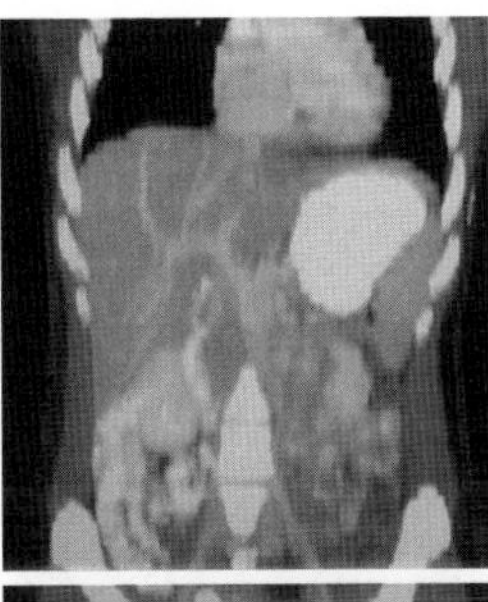
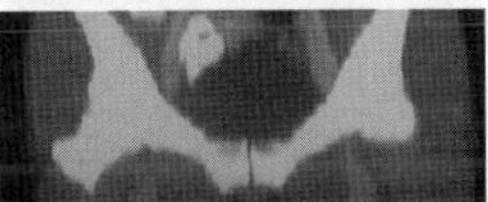

Portal Venous Phase

1. sigmoid colon
2. cecum
3. terminal ileum
4. iliac wing
5. gluteus medius muscle
6. gluteus maximus muscle

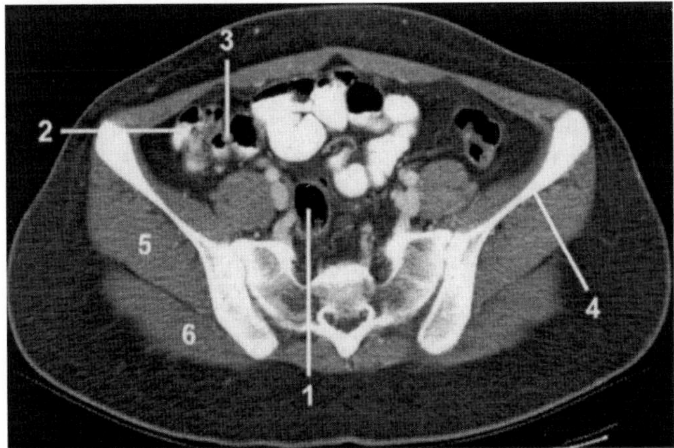

Portal Venous Phase

1. sigmoid colon
2. cecum
3. vermiform appendix
4. gluteus medius
5. gluteus maximus
6. internal iliac art and vein

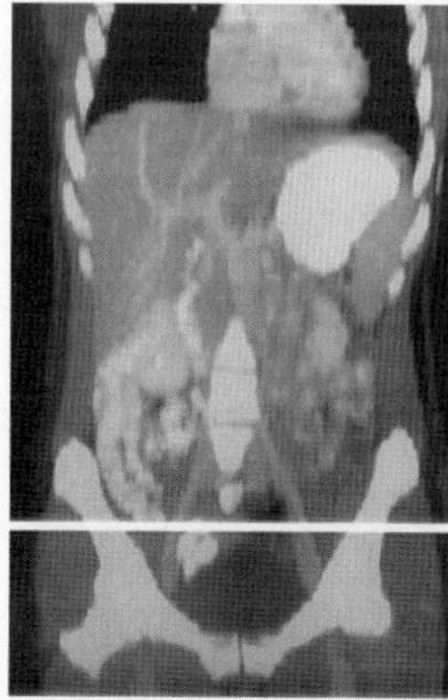

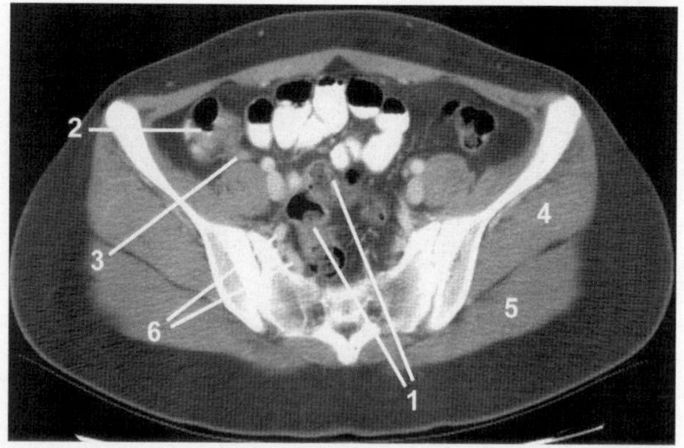

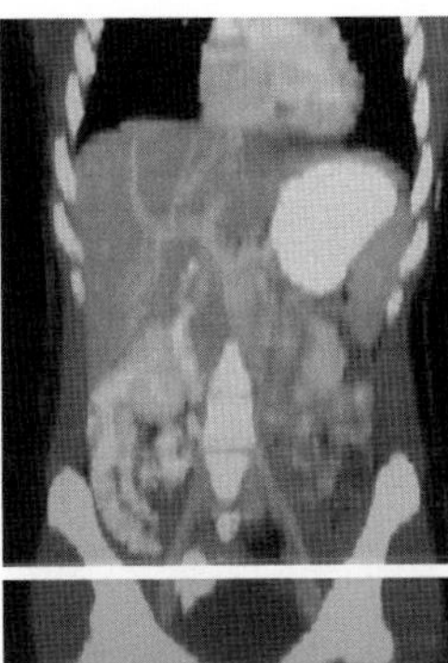

Portal Venous Phase

1. external iliac art
2. external iliac vein
3. left sacroiliac joint
4. sigmoid colon
5. gluteus maximus muscle
6. gluteus medius muscle
7. gluteus minimus muscle

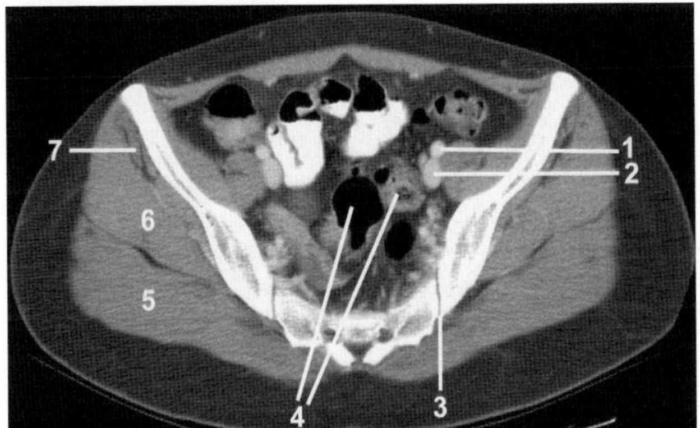

Female

1. right ovary
2. sigmoid colon
3. piriformis muscle
4. iliacus muscle
5. psoas muscle

UT, uterus (fundus)

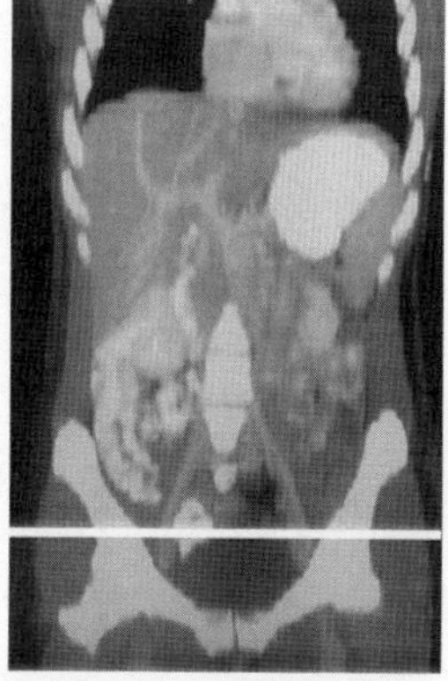

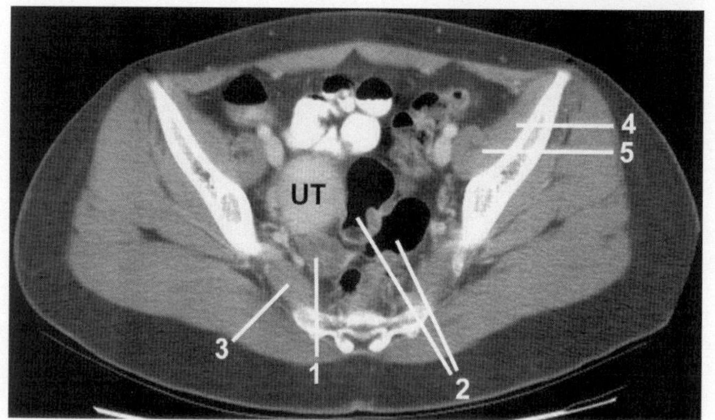

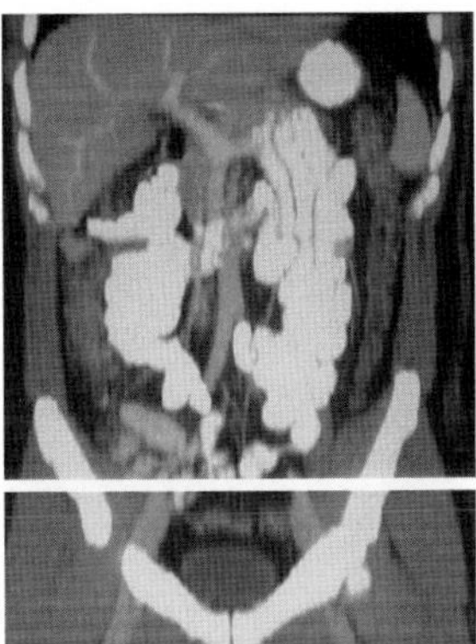

Male

1. gluteus maximus muscle
2. gluteus medius muscle
3. gluteus minimus muscle
4. iliopsoas muscle
5. small bowel loops

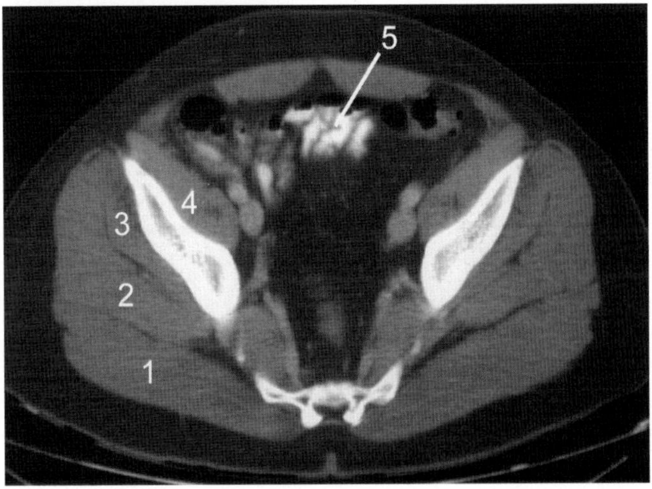

Female

1. left ovary
2. physiologic fluid in pelvis (normal in menstruating-age female)
3. uterine fundus
4. endometrial cavity
5. iliopsoas muscle
6. gluteus minimus muscle
7. gluteus medius muscle
8. gluteus maximus muscle

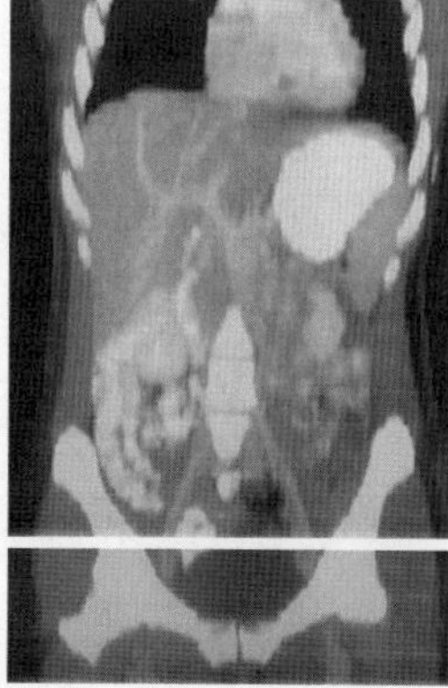

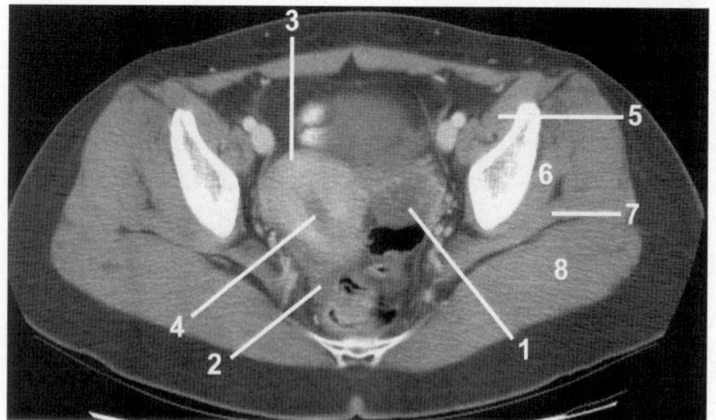

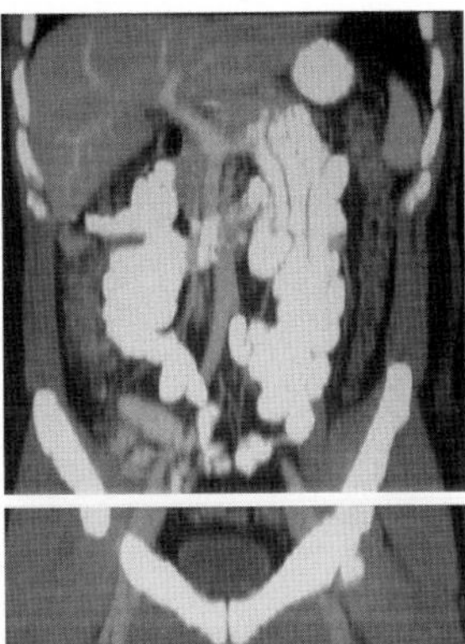

Male

1. sigmoid colon
2. gluteus maximus muscle
3. gluteus medius muscle
4. gluteus minimus muscle
5. iliopsoas muscle
6. piriformis muscle

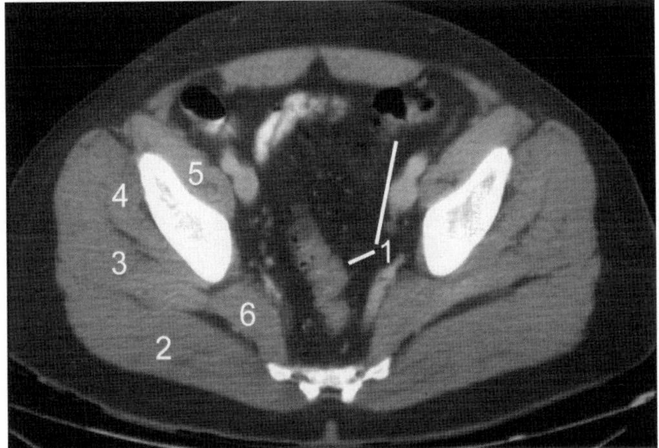

Female

1. left ovary
2. physiologic free fluid (normal in menstruating-age female)
3. uterus (endometrial cavity)
4. iliopsoas muscle
5. rectum
6. round ligament of uterus

UB, urinary bladder

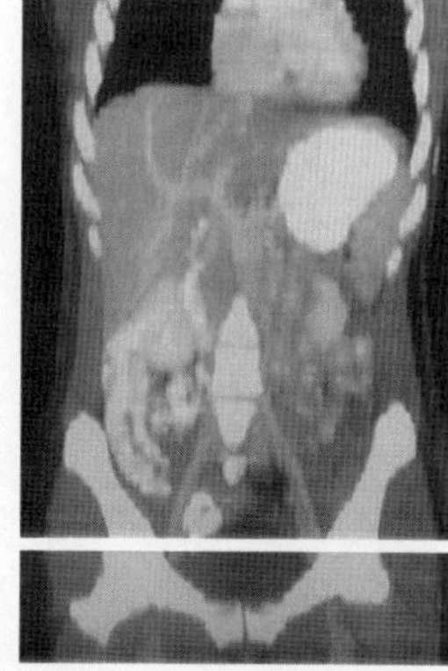

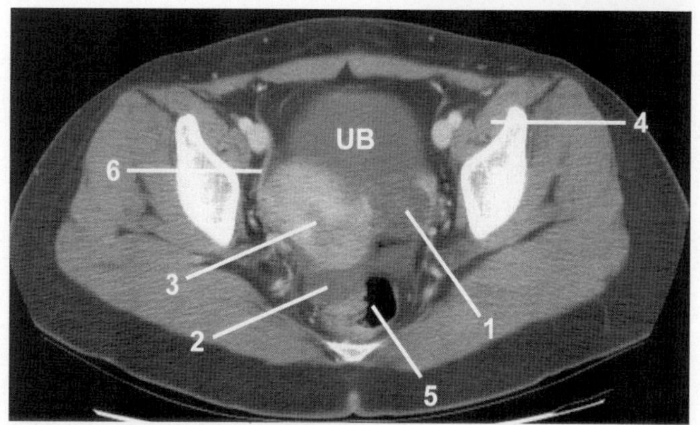

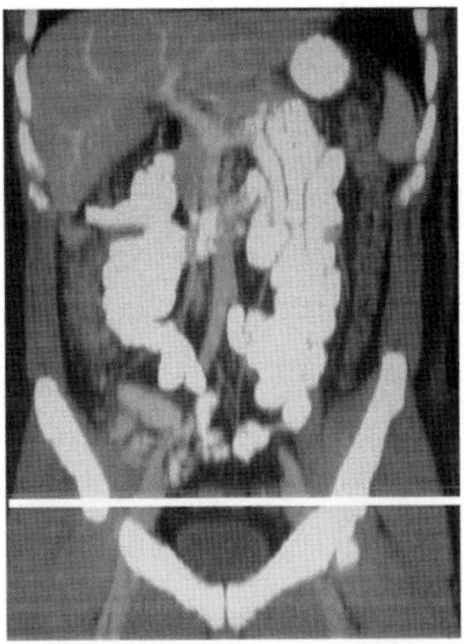

Male

1. sigmoid colon
2. iliopsoas muscle
3. rectus abdominus muscle
4. obturator internus muscle
5. acetabular roof

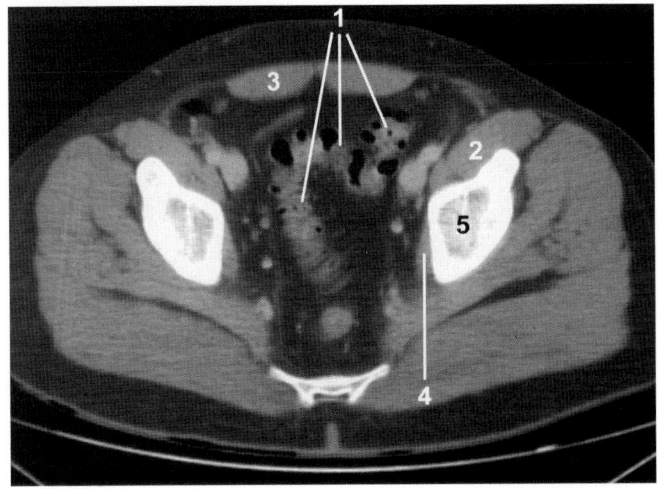

Female

1. rectum
2. uterine cervix
3. iliopsoas muscle
4. obturator internus muscle
5. acetabular roof

UB, urinary bladder

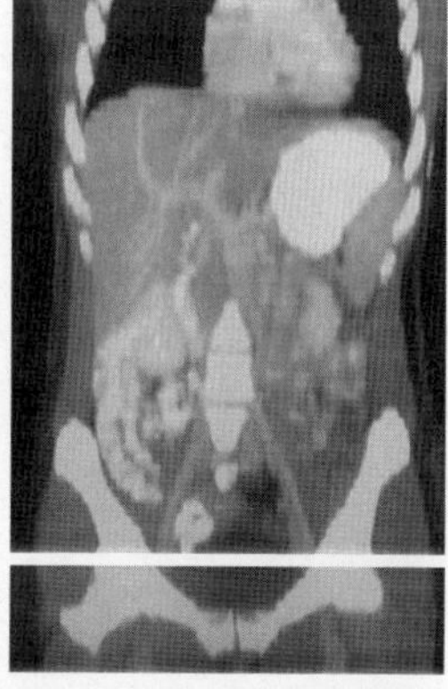

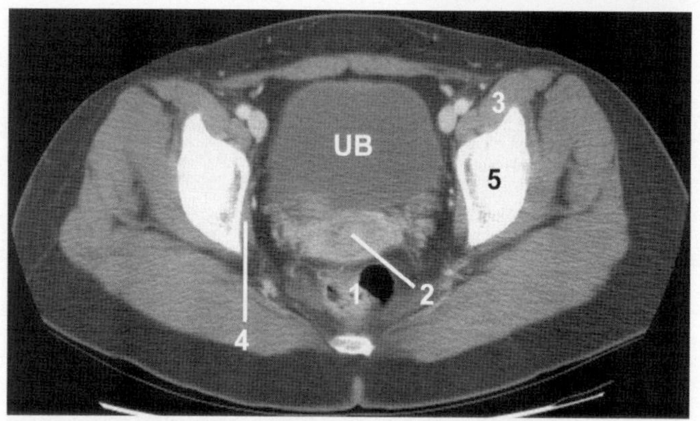

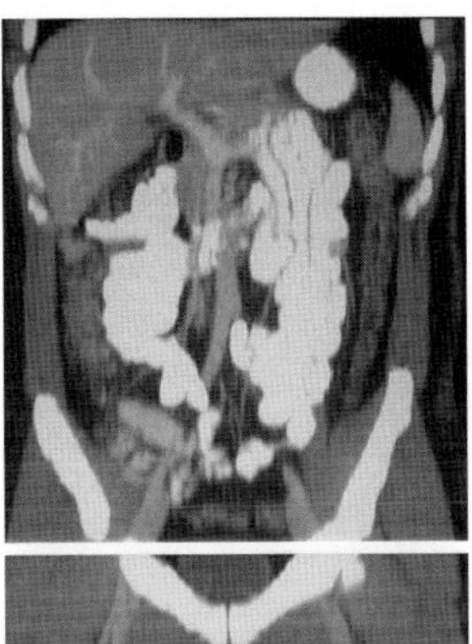

Male

1. external iliac vein
2. external iliac art
3. gluteus maximus muscle
4. gluteus medius muscle
5. gluteus minimus muscle
6. iliopsoas muscle
7. obturator internus muscle

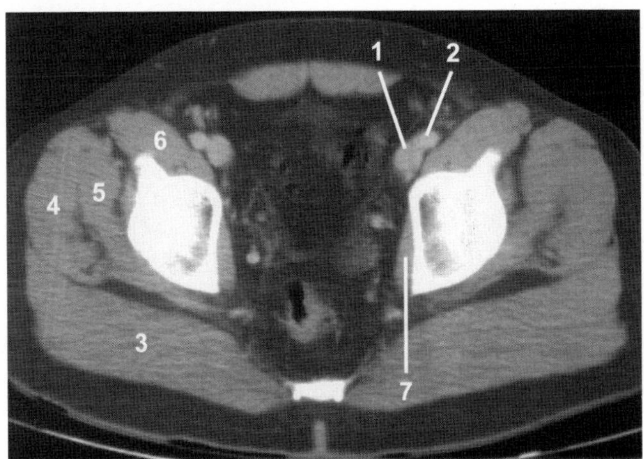

Female

1. uterine cervix
2. femoral head
3. ant acetabulum
4. post acetabulum

UB, urinary bladder

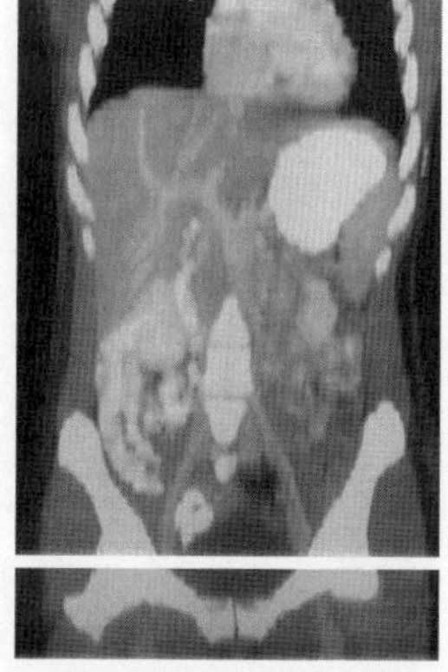

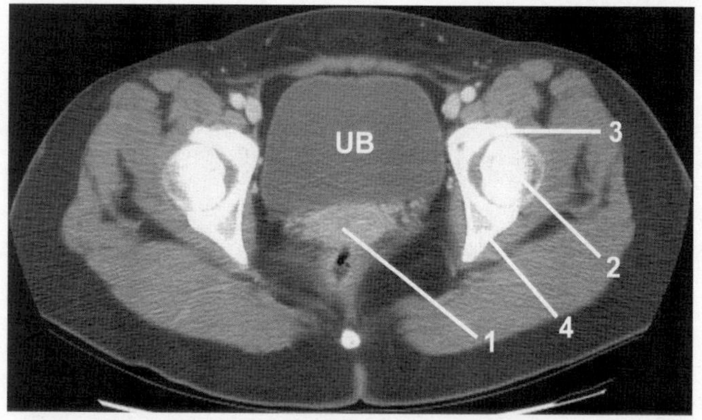

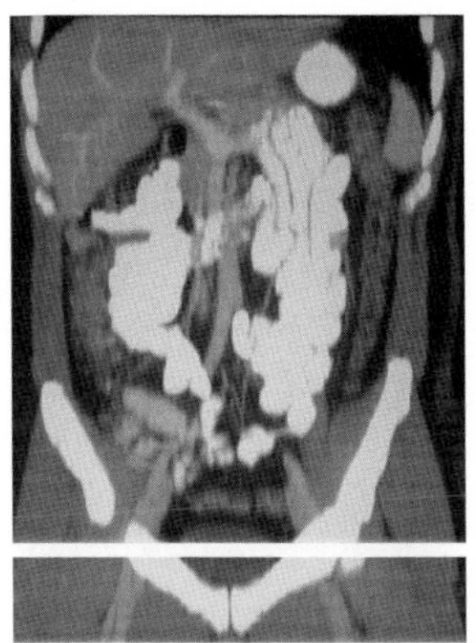

Male

1. seminal vesicles
2. rectum

UB, urinary bladder

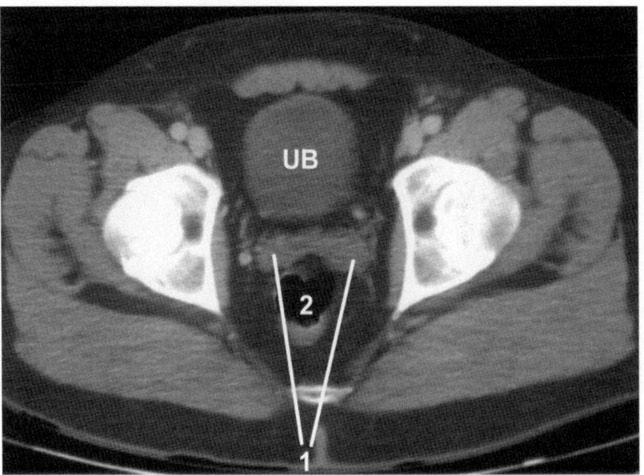

Female

1. anus
2. tip of coccyx
3. obturator internus muscle
4. greater trochanter of femur
5. vagina
6. ischiorectal fossa
7. common femoral art
8. common femoral vein
9. femoral head

UB, urinary bladder

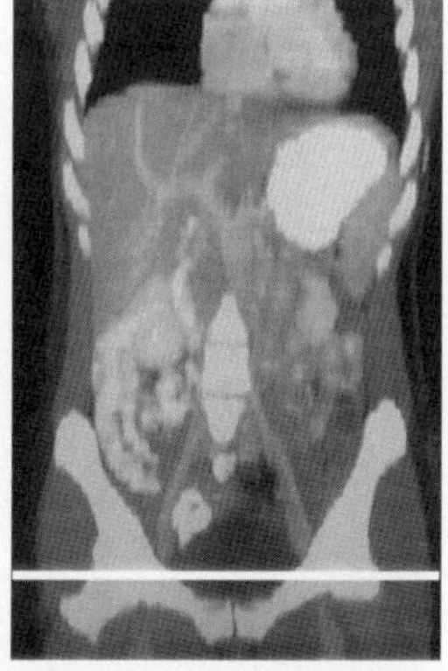

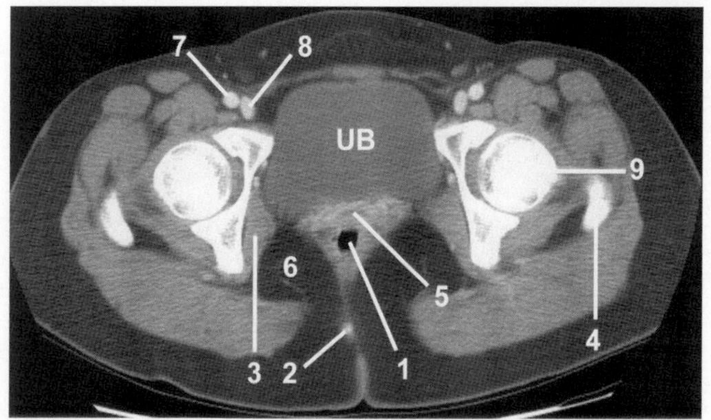

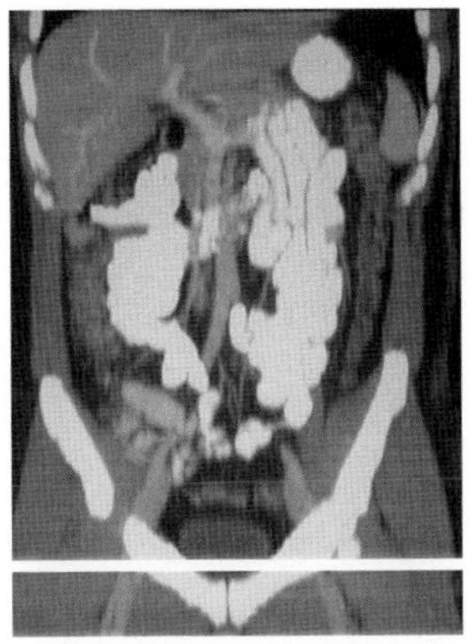

Male

1. femur
2. prostate
3. rectum
4. levator ani muscle

UB, urinary bladder

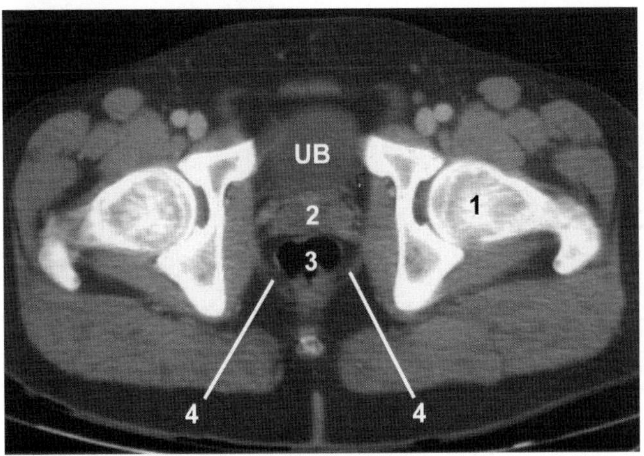

Female

1. anus
2. vagina
3. obturator internus muscle
4. iliopsoas muscle
5. rectus femoris muscle
6. tensor fasciae latae muscle
7. sartorius muscle
8. vastus lateralis muscle
9. ischium

UB, urinary bladder

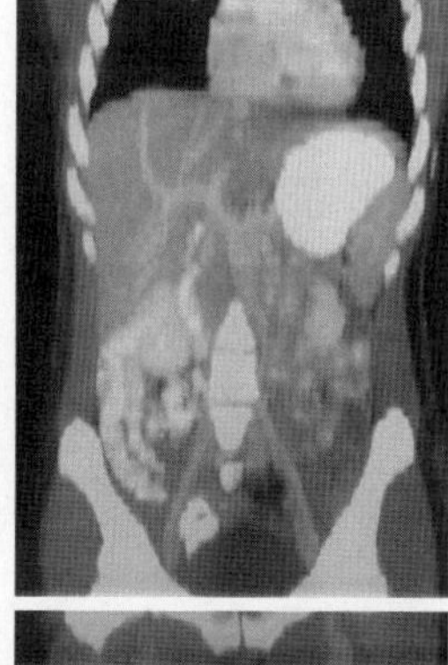

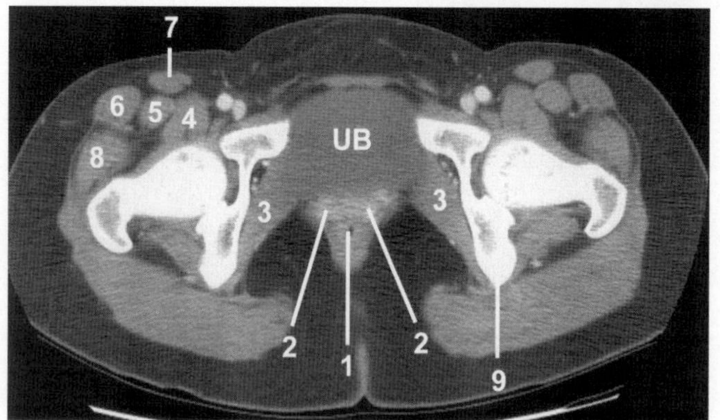

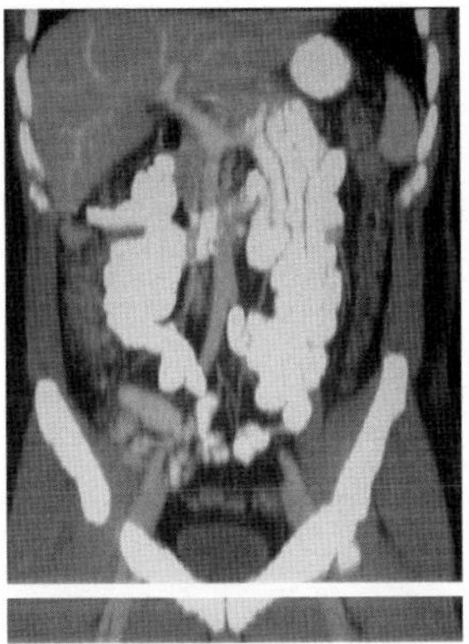

Male

1. prostate
2. rectum
3. obturator internus muscle
4. spermatic cords

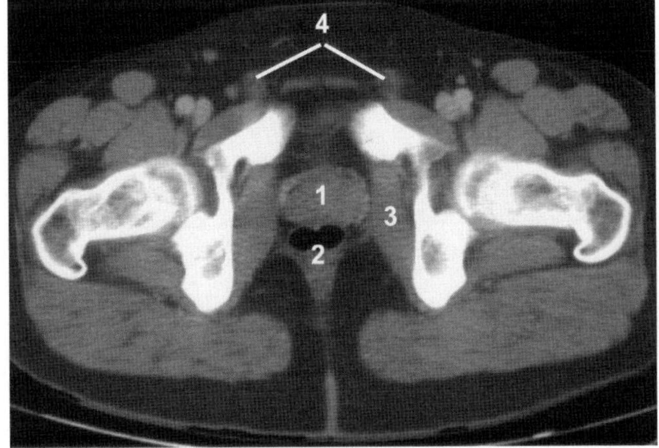

Female

1. obturator externus muscle
2. pectineus muscle
3. symphysis pubis
4. ischium
5. neck of femur
6. superior pubic ramus

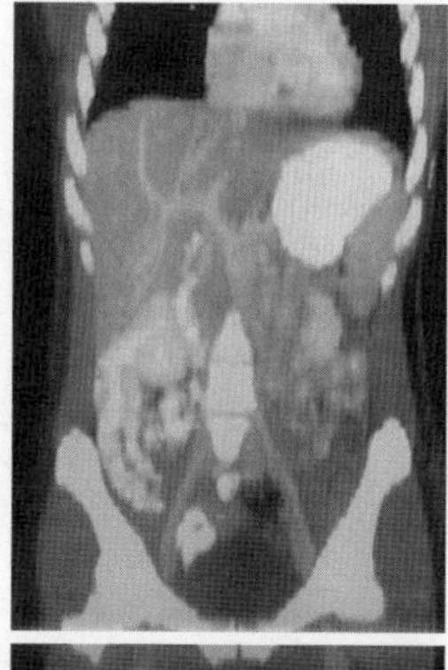

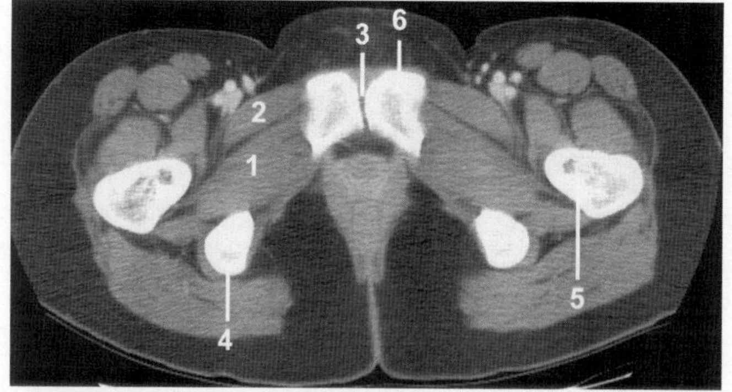

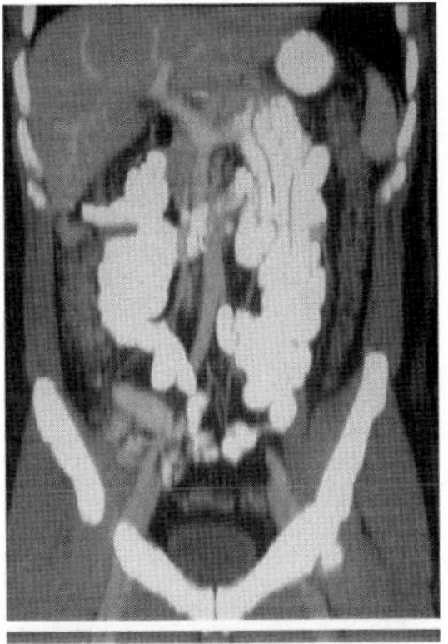

Male

1. prostate
2. rectum
3. levator ani muscle
4. pectineus muscle
5. obturator externus muscle
6. obturator internus muscle

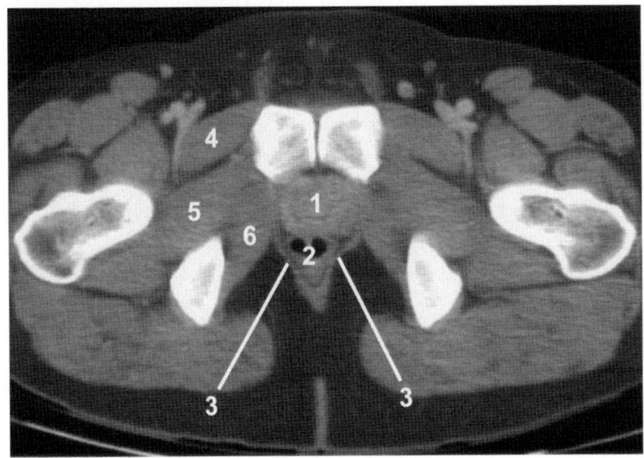

Female

1. inferior pubic ramus
2. pectineus muscle
3. iliopsoas muscle
4. ischiorectal fossa

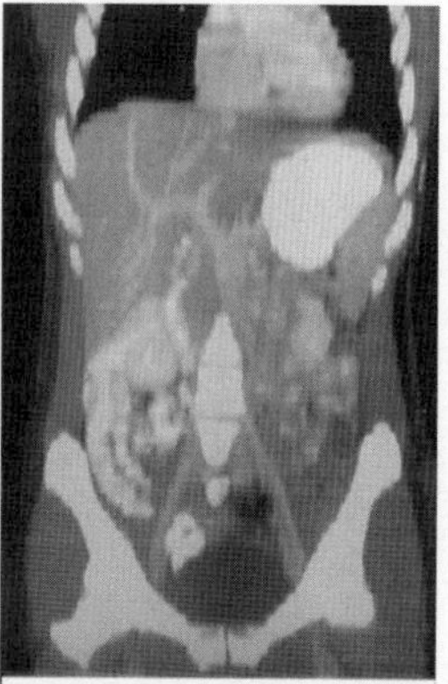

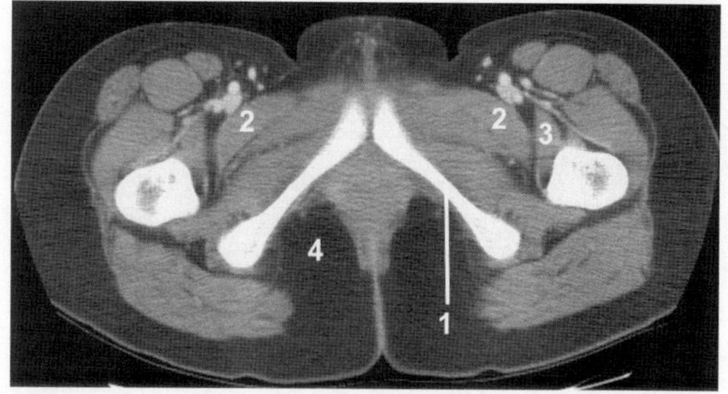

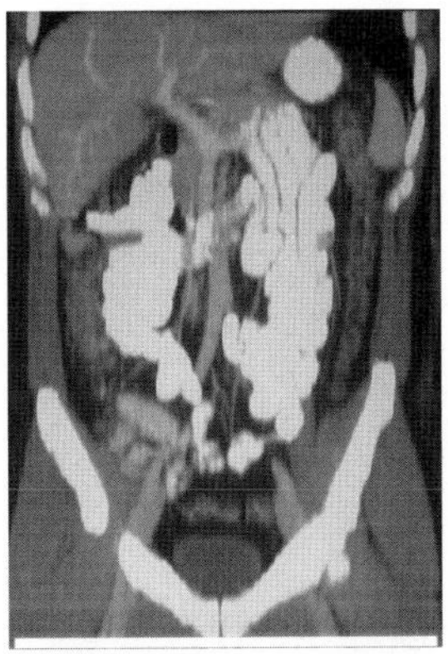

Male

1. rectum
2. inferior pubic ramus
3. ischiorectal fossa
4. iliopsoas muscle
5. rectus femoris muscle
6. sartorius muscle
7. tensor fasciae latae muscle
8. vastus lateralis muscle
9. spermatic cord
10. corpora cavernosa of penis

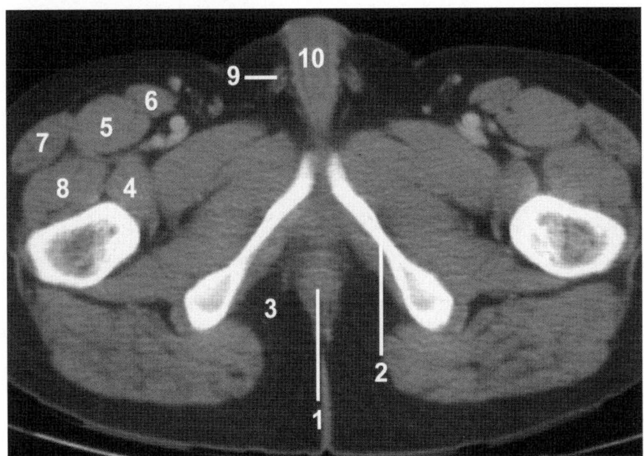

Abdomen, Arterial Phase

Abdomen, Arterial Phase/Axial

1. caudate lobe of liver
2. main portal vein
3. inferior vena cava
4. left diaphragmatic crus

A, abdominal aorta
RL Liver, right lobe of liver
Spl, spleen
Stom, stomach

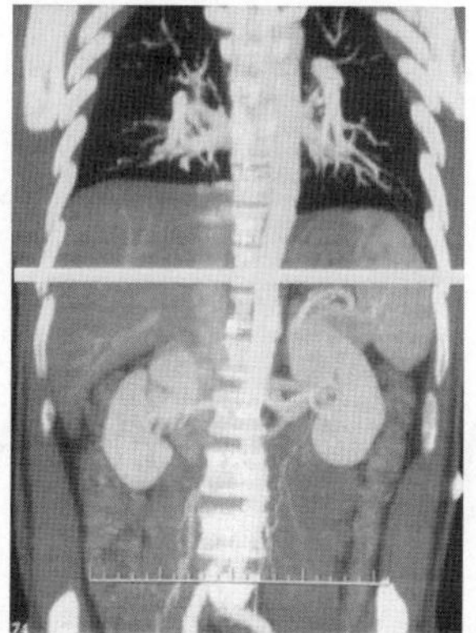

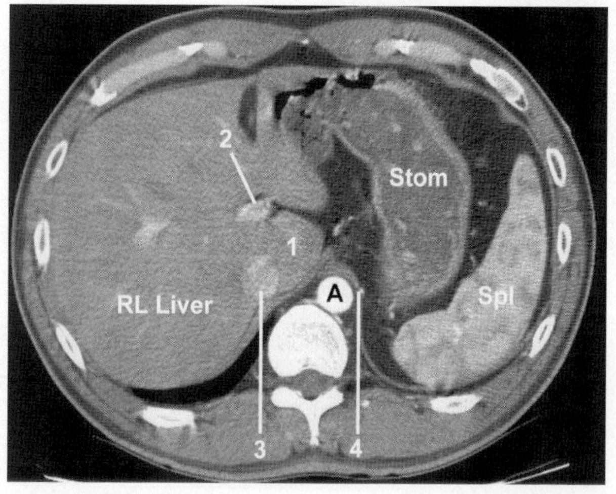

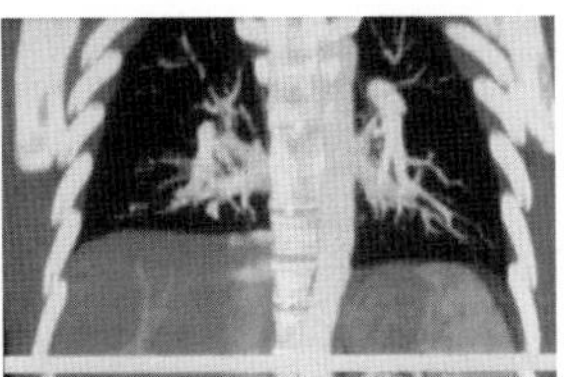

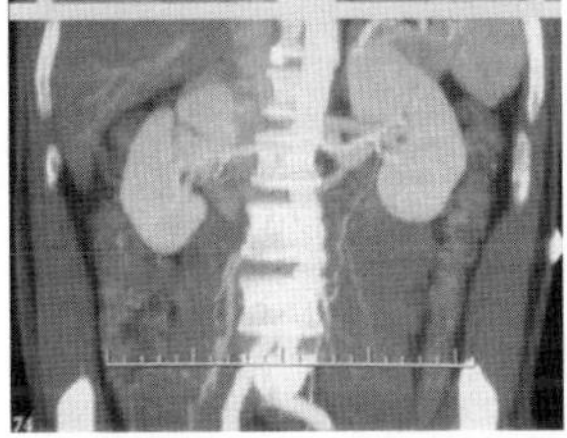

1. hepatic art
2. splenic flexure
3. splenic art
4. pancreas
5. inferior vena cava
6. main portal vein
7. left adrenal gland
8. left gastric art

A, abdominal aorta
Antrum, antrum of stomach
RL Liver, right lobe of liver
Spl, spleen

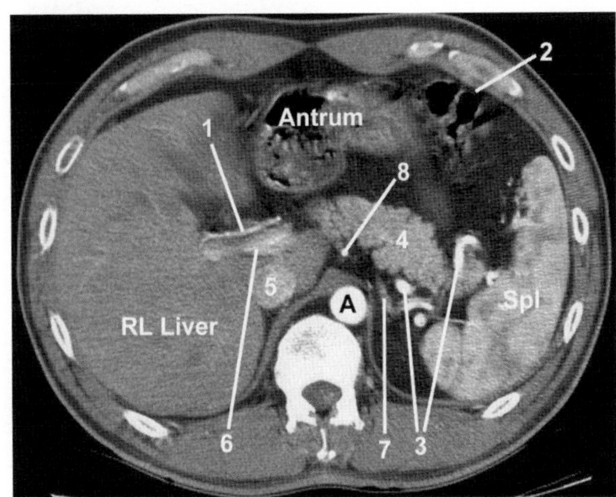

Abdomen, Arterial Phase/Axial

1. splenic art
2. splenic flexure
3. inferior vena cava
4. pancreas (body)
5. adrenal glands
6. gastroduodenal art

A, abdominal aorta
Ant, antrum of stomach
GB, gallbladder
Spl, spleen

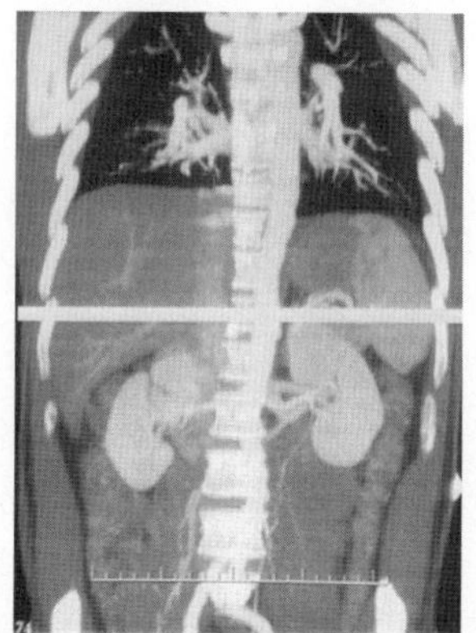

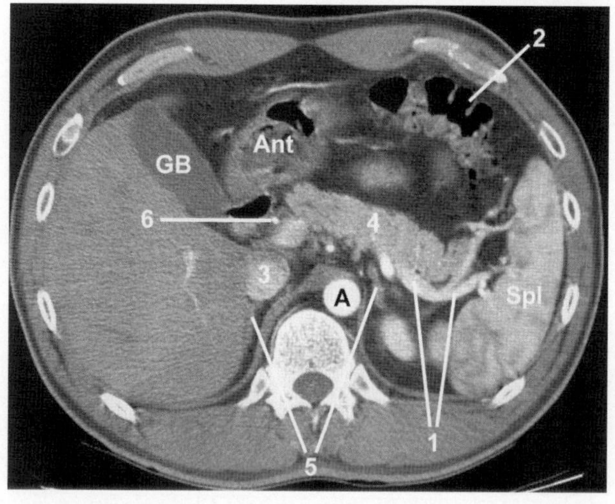

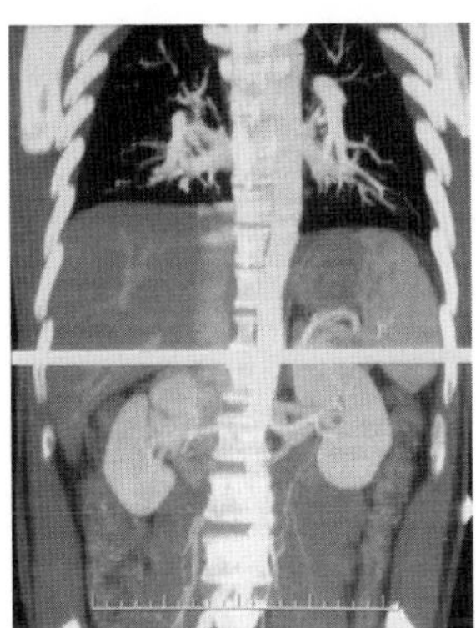

1. splenic art
2. celiac art
3. splenic flexure of colon
4. pancreas (tail)
5. adrenal glands
6. gastroduodenal art
7. duodenum (bulb)
8. gallbladder
9. portosplenic vein confluence

Spl, spleen

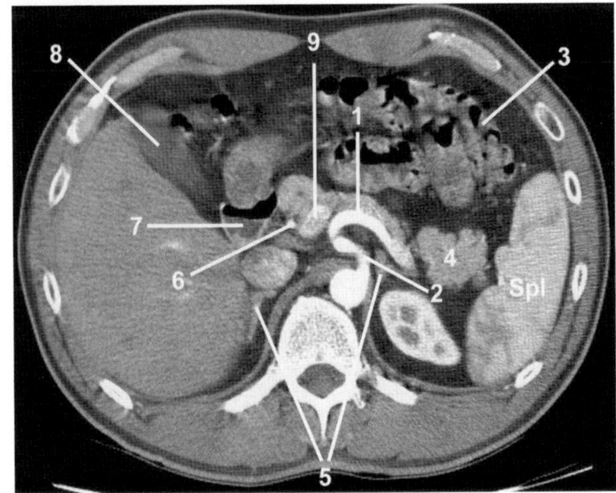

1. gastroduodenal art
2. duodenum
3. splenic vein
4. portosplenic vein confluence
5. erector spinae muscles
6. adrenal glands
7. inferior vena cava
8. transverse colon
9. adrenal glands

A, abdominal aorta
LK, left kidney
Spl, spleen

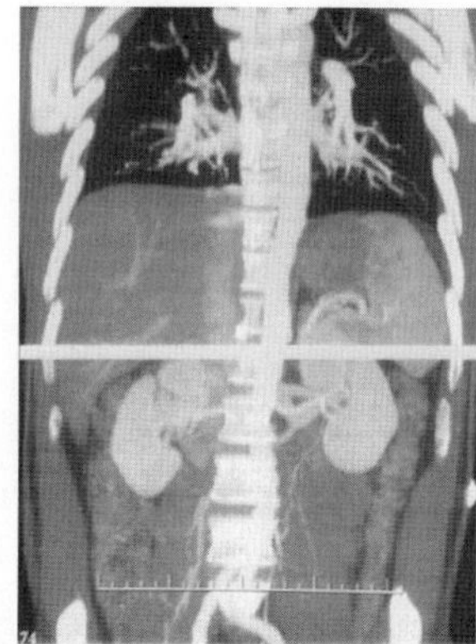

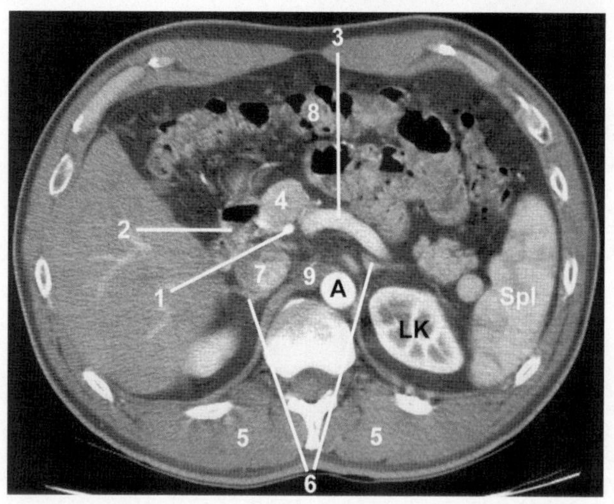

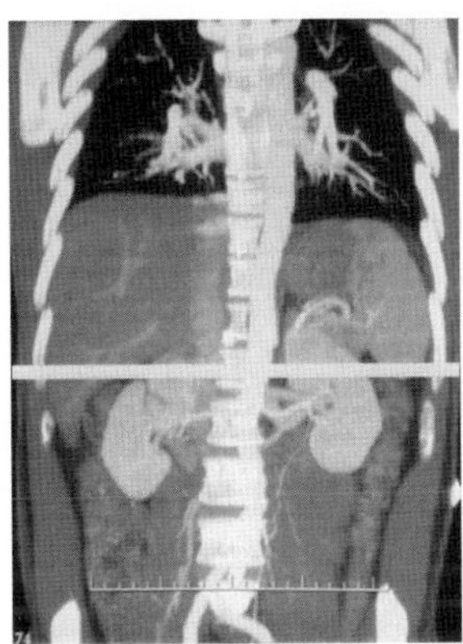

1. superior mesenteric art
2. inferior vena cava
3. right lobe of liver
4. pancreas (head)
5. crus of diaphragm
6. transverse colon

LK, left kidney
RK, right kidney
Spl, spleen

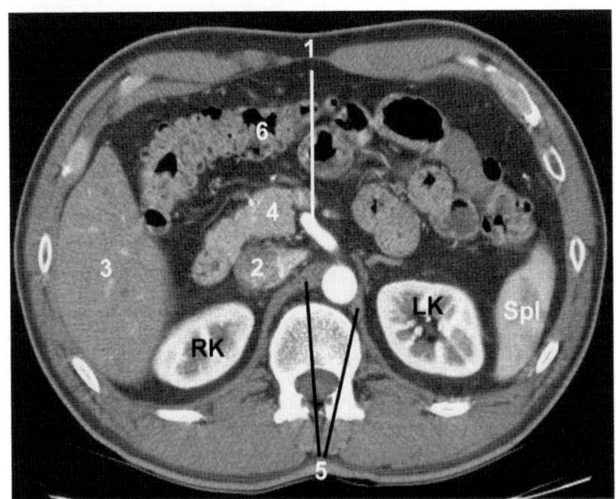

1. superior mesenteric art
2. inferior vena cava
3. duodenum (descending)
4. pancreas (head)
5. left renal vein

A, abdominal aorta
J, jejunal loops
LK, left kidney
RK, right kidney

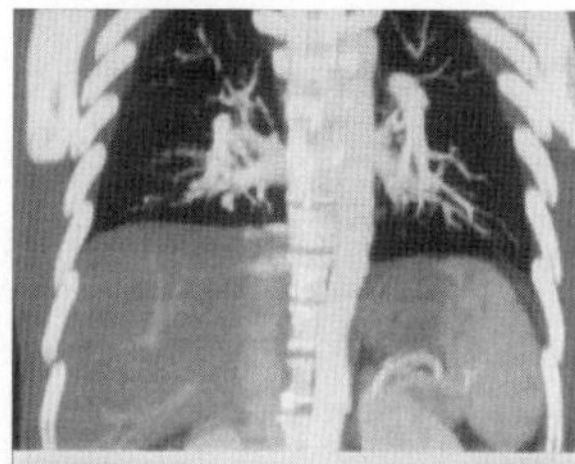

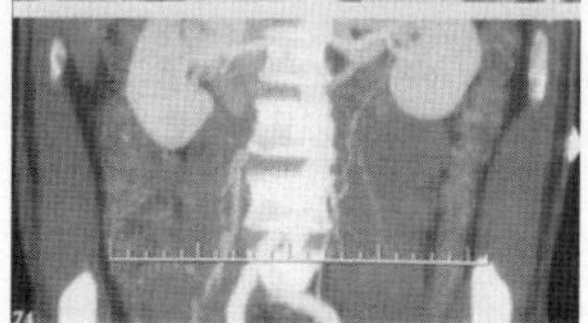

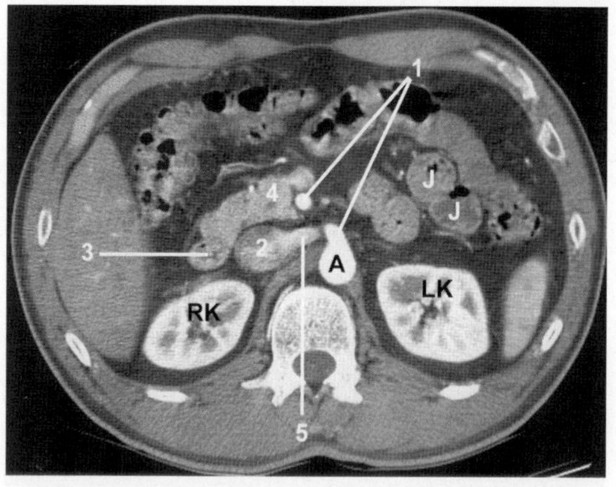

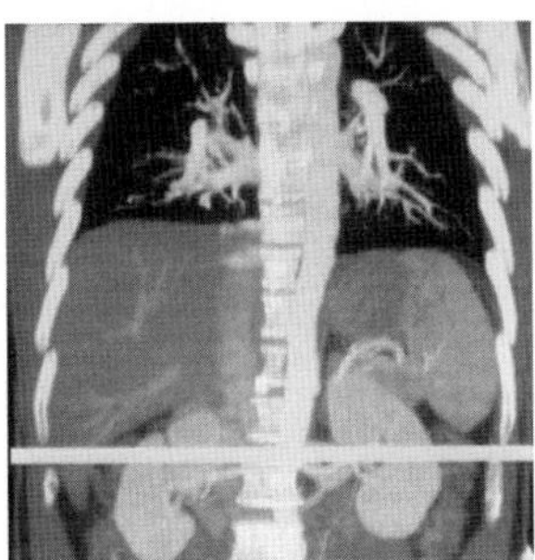

1. inferior vena cava
2. duodenum
3. superior mesenteric art
4. left renal vein
5. right lobe of liver

J, jejunum
LK, left kidney
Om, omental fat
RK, right kidney

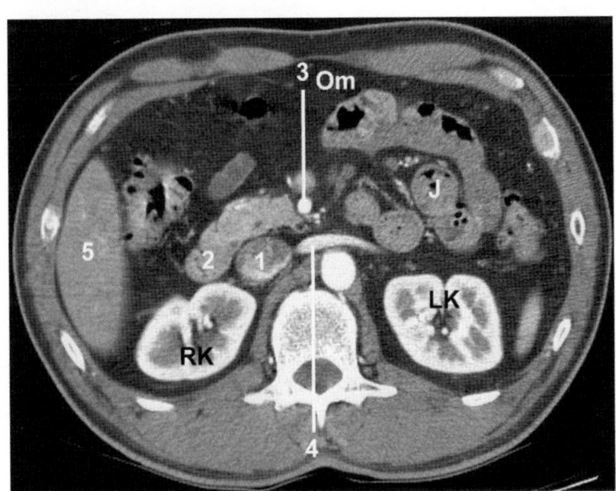

Abdomen, Arterial Phase/Axial

1. duodenum
2. pancreas (head)
3. right renal art
4. left renal vein
5. inferior vena cava
6. superior mesenteric art
7. crus of diaphragm

A, abdominal aorta
AC, ascending colon
DC, descending colon
J, jejunum
LK, left kidney
RK, right kidney

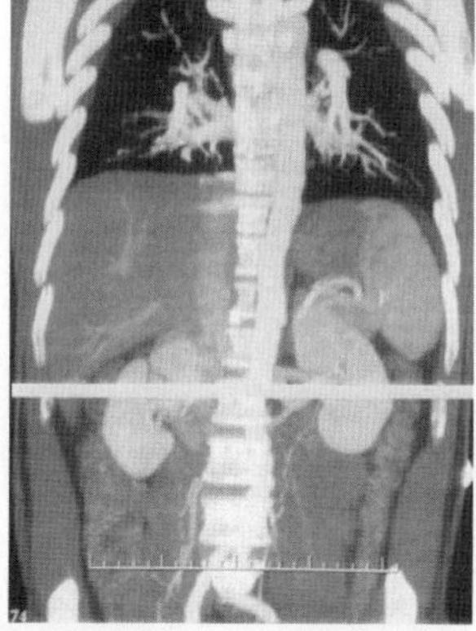

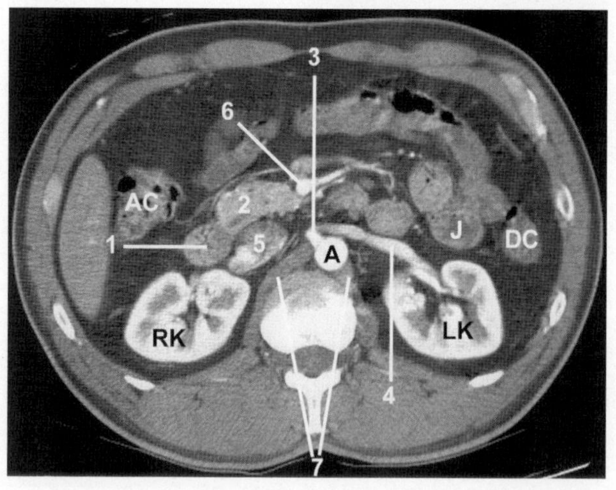

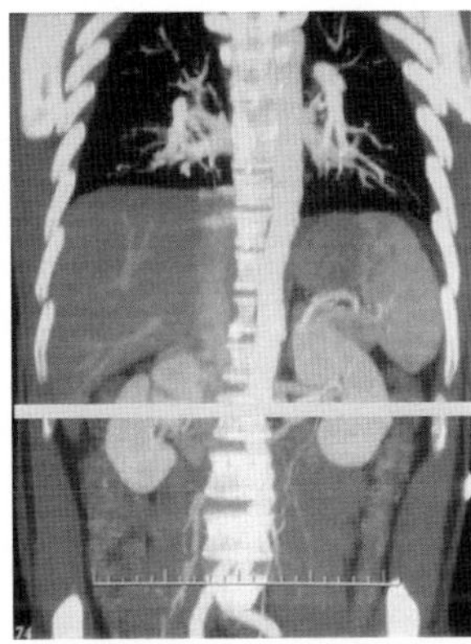

1. right renal vein
2. left renal art
3. right renal art
4. inferior vena cava
5. rectus abdominus muscles

A, abdominal aorta
AC, ascending colon
D, duodenum
DC, descending colon
LK, left kidney
RK, right kidney

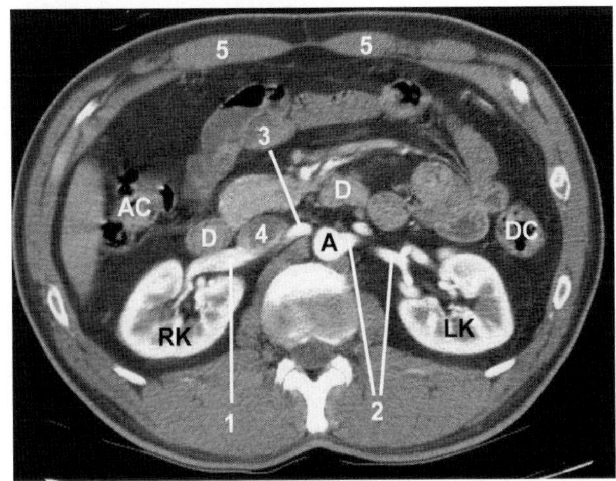

1. pancreas
2. inferior vena cava
3. right renal art
4. left renal art
5. right renal vein

AC, ascending colon
DC, descending colon
J, jejunal loops
L, liver tip
LK, left kidney
RK, right kidney

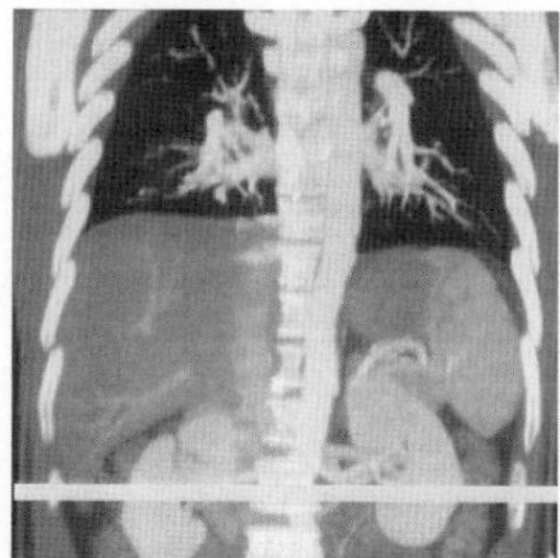

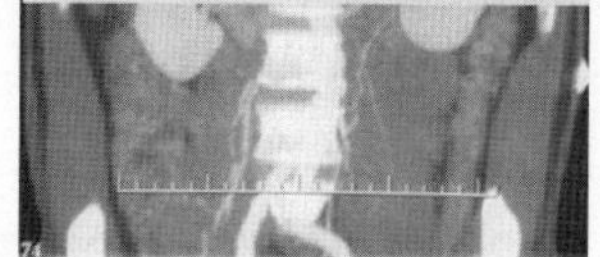

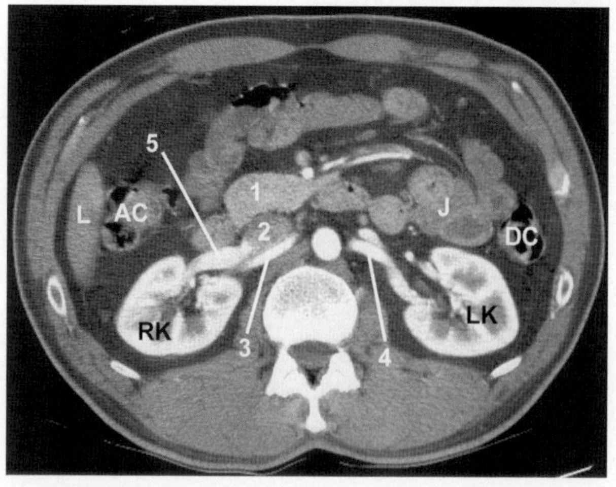

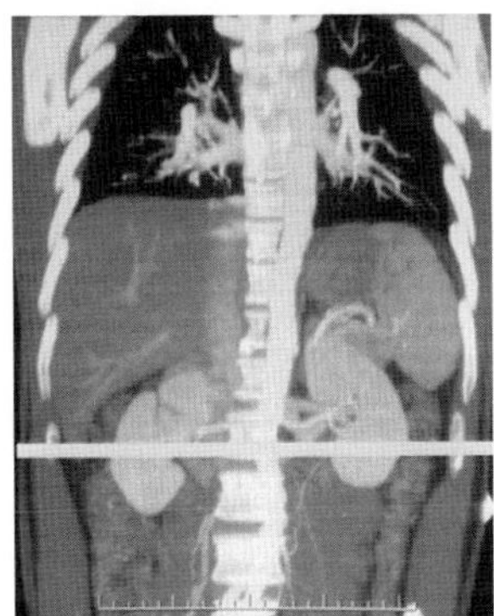

1. duodenum
2. inferior vena cava
3. quadratus lumborum muscles
4. rectus abdominus muscles

A, abdominal aorta
AC, ascending colon
DC, descending colon
J, jejunum
LK, left kidney
Ps, psoas muscles
RK, right kidney

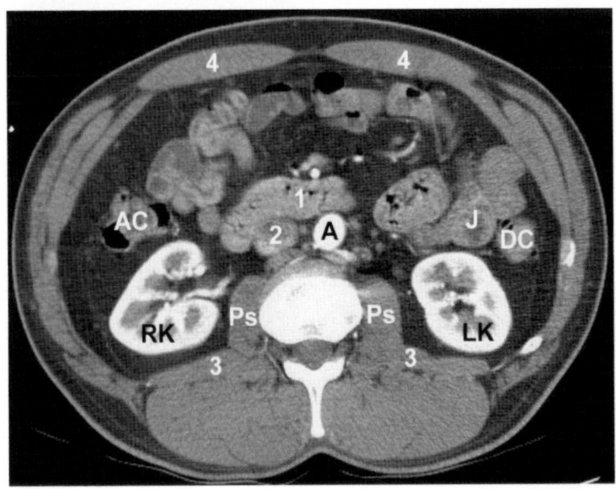

Abdomen and Pelvis Reconstructions

Arterial Phase Coronal Maximum Intensity Projection Image

1. left renal art
2. right renal art
3. left common iliac art

A, abdominal aorta
AC, ascending colon
DC, descending colon
Liv, liver
LK, left kidney
RK, right kidney
Spl, spleen
Stom, stomach

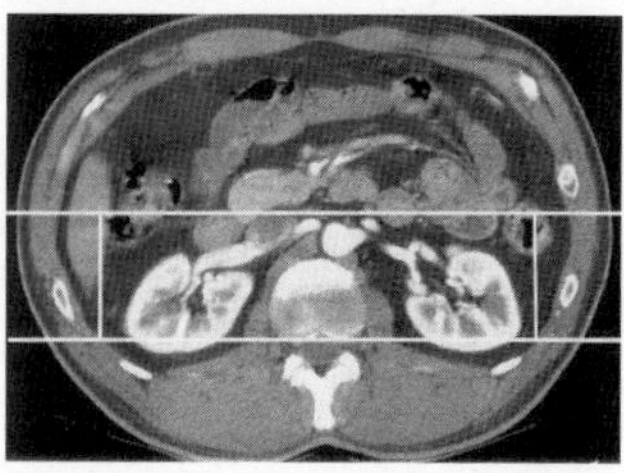

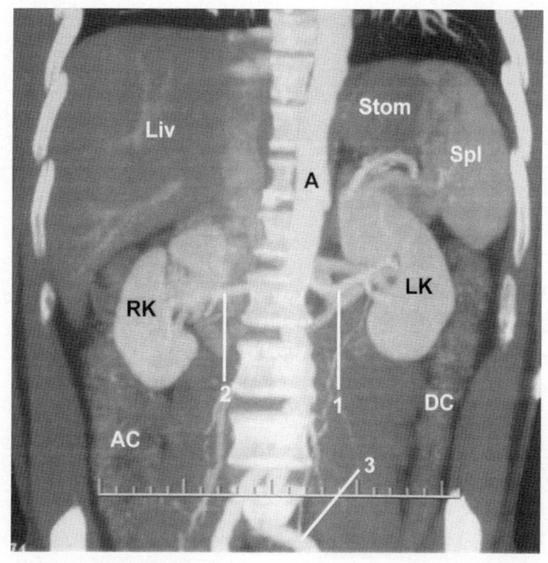

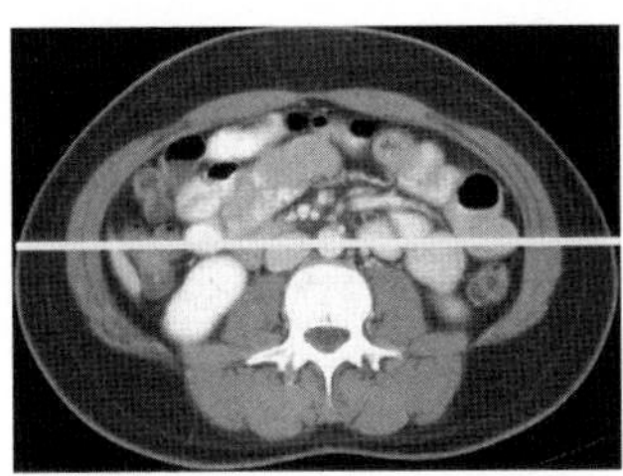

Coronal Abdomen

1. left iliac bone
2. main portal vein
3. inferior vena cava
4. ascending colon
5. descending colon

A, abdominal aorta
Liv, liver
Ps, psoas muscle
Spl, spleen
Stom, stomach
UB, urinary bladder

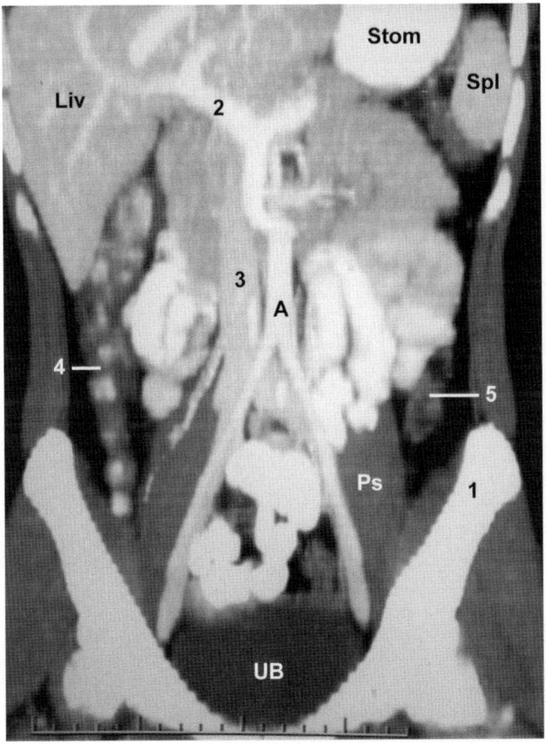

Abdominal Aorta: Volume Rendering

1. left gastric art
2. common hepatic art
3. proper hepatic art
4. gastroduodenal art
5. splenic art
6. superior mesenteric art
7. left renal art
8. celiac art

A, abdominal aorta
LK, left kidney
RK, right kidney

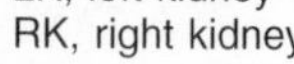

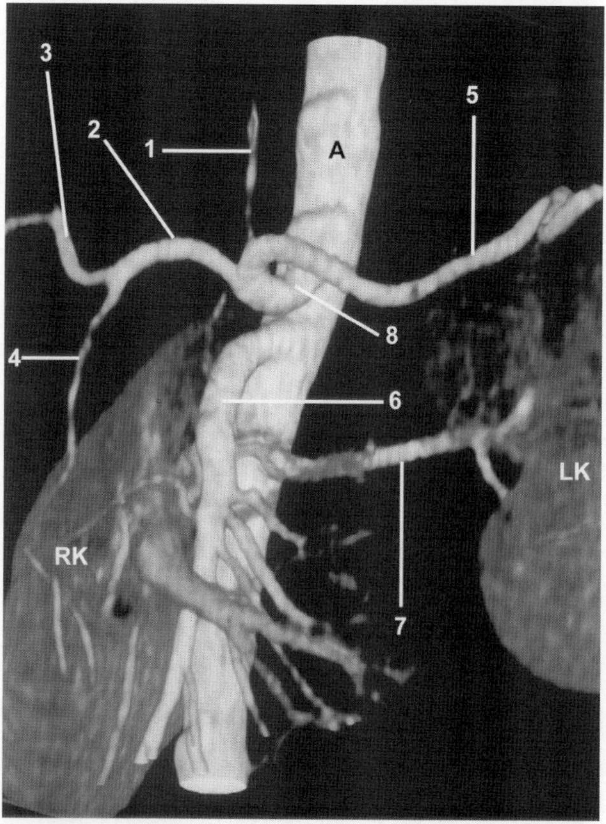